Praise for

the mindful path to self-compassion

"In this important book, Christopher Germer illuminates the myriad synergies between mindfulness and compassion. He offers skillful and effective ways of making sure that we are inviting ourselves to bathe in and benefit from the kind heart of awareness itself, and from the actions that follow from such a radical and sane embrace."

—Jon Kabat-Zinn, PhD, author of *Arriving at Your Own Door* and *Letting Everything Become Your Teacher*

"Self-compassion is the ground of all emotional healing, and Dr. Germer has produced an invaluable guide. Written with great clarity, psychological wisdom, and warmth, this book will serve anyone seeking practical and powerful tools that free the heart."

—Tara Brach, PhD, author of *Radical Acceptance*

"Explains both the science and practice of developing kindness toward ourselves and others. Dr. Germer offers powerful and easily accessible steps toward transforming our lives from the inside out. It's never too late to start along this important path."

—Daniel J. Siegel, MD, author of *The Mindful Brain*

"An elegant and practical guide to cultivating self-compassion, by a dedicated and wise clinician and meditation teacher. The author offers time-honored practices and exercises with the potential to illuminate and transform the background chatter of our minds that determines so much of the course of our lives."

—Samuel Shem, MD, author of *The House of God*

the mindful path to self-compassion

Freeing Yourself from Destructive Thoughts and Emotions

CHRISTOPHER K. GERMER, PhD

Foreword by Sharon Salzberg

THE GUILFORD PRESS
New York   London

Library of Congress Cataloging-in-Publication Data
Germer, Christopher K.
     The mindful path to self-compassion : freeing yourself from
  destructive thoughts and emotions / Christopher K. Germer. —
  1st ed.
          p.   cm.
     Includes bibliographical references and index.
     ISBN 978-1-60623-284-2 (hardcover : alk. paper) —
  ISBN 978-1-59385-975-6 (pbk. : alk. paper)
     1. Emotions. 2. Compassion. 3. Thought and
  thinking. 4. Meditations—Therapeutic use.   I. Title.
     BF531.G47 2009
     152'.4—dc22
                                                2008054860

To my mother,
who taught me the meaning of compassion

contents

Part III
customizing self-compassion

foreword

Why is it so hard to extend the same kindness to ourselves that many of us gladly offer to others? Maybe it's because in our conventional way of thinking in the West we tend to view compassion as a gift, and bestowing it on ourselves seems selfish or inappropriate. But the ancient wisdom of the East tells us that loving-kindness is something everyone needs and deserves, and that includes the compassion we can give to ourselves. Without it, we blame ourselves for our problems, for our inability to solve them all, for feeling pain when painful events occur—all of which usually end in our feeling even more pain.

The idea of self-compassion may seem so alien that we would not know where to begin even if we decided it might be a good capacity to develop. Modern neuroscience and psychology are just beginning to explore what meditative traditions have accepted for ages: that compassion and loving-kindness are *skills*—not gifts that we're either born with or not—and each one of us, without exception, can develop and strengthen these skills and bring them into our everyday lives.

This is where *The Mindful Path to Self-Compassion* steps to the fore. In this book Dr. Christopher Germer lays out the architecture of this skill development: the vision of freedom compassion can offer, the essential role of self-compassion, the path to realizing it rather than just thinking about it, and the practical tools, such as mindfulness, we need to effect that transformation.

Buddhist psychological analysis regards qualities like loving-kindness as the direct antidote to fear. Whether hampered by the inhibiting fear of feeling we are not enough and could never be enough, or the raging fear that courses through us when we see no options whatsoever, or the pervasive fear we sometimes feel when we must take a next step and cannot sense how or where, in the midst of fear we suffer. Loving-kindness and compassion, in contrast to fear, reaffirm the healing power of connection, the expansiveness of a sense of possibility, the efficacy of kindness as a catalyst for learning. Whether extended to ourselves or others, the intertwined forces of loving-kindness and compassion are the basis for wise, powerful, sometimes gentle, and sometimes fierce actions that can really make a difference—in our own lives and those of others. The true development of self-compassion is the basis for fearlessness, generosity, inclusion, and a sustained loving-kindness and compassion for others.

Whether you have already begun to seek relief from suffering through meditative traditions like mindfulness or you are simply open to anything that might free you from chronic emotional pain and mental rumination, this book will serve as an inspiring roadmap. In the following pages you will find a scientific review, an educational manual, and a practical step-by-step guide to developing greater loving-kindness and self-compassion every day.

SHARON SALZBERG
Insight Meditation Society, Barre, Massachusetts

acknowledgments

Writing can be lonely work, but with so many people speaking through the pages of this book, that's hardly been the case. I had the privilege of gathering the voices of kindness and inspiration that have been resonating in my mind for a long time—teachers, family, friends, patients—and savored their company late into the night for almost two years. Now that the project is completed, it's a privilege to mention some of them by name.

First I'd like to thank my wonderful team of editors at The Guilford Press: Kitty Moore, Linda Carbone, and Chris Benton. Kitty's faith in the project, editorial style, and practical wisdom transformed a nascent idea into reality. Linda's graceful editing lifted this manuscript to its current level of readability, and Chris's conceptual clarity gave the book its overall coherence and flow. If these dedicated people weren't editors, they'd be coauthors.

My friends and colleagues at the Institute for Meditation and Psychotherapy have been invaluable, not only in shaping the content of this book but also in their unstinting emotional support. It's been a family affair in the best sense of the word. My brothers and sisters include Paul Fulton, Trudy Goodman, Sara Lazar, Bill and Susan Morgan, Stephanie Morgan, Andrew Olendzki, Tom Pedulla, Susan Pollak, Ron Siegel, Charles Styron, and Jan Surrey. I'm especially indebted to Sara for her advice on all things scientific, to Andy for anchoring my thinking in the 2,500-year-old tradition of Buddhist psychology, to Ron for keeping it real, to Jan for her exquisite and abiding sense of interconnection, and to Trudy for lending a touch of bold tenderness to the subject matter.

My personal practice of self-compassion has been inspired by the writings and presence of a number of special teachers. They are His Holiness the Dalai Lama, Sharon Salzberg, Jon Kabat-Zinn, Tara Brach, Pema Chödrön, Joseph Goldstein, Jack Kornfield, and Thich Nhat Hanh. Furthermore, my understanding of self-compassion would be nowhere if not for the groundbreaking work of my friend and colleague Kristin Neff and researchers Paul Gilbert and Mark Leary, and for the bold new understanding of therapeutic change by Mark Epstein, Steven Hayes, Marsha Linehan, Zindel Siegel, and their collaborators. Thanks also to Richard Davidson, Daniel Goleman, and Daniel Siegel for inspiring me and countless other readers around the world to look at human emotion and interpersonal relationships from a profoundly unselfish, scientific perspective.

Other friends and colleagues who made this book possible were Jay Efran, for teaching me in graduate school that all psychological theories are provisional; Les Havens, for demonstrating the importance of being human in psychotherapy; Rich Simon, for his encouragement and gentle writing lessons; Robert and Barry, for the best writing fuel this side of the Charles River; Carol Hosmer, for keeping my practice running; Rob Guerette, for taking a chance on mindfulness and self-compassion; and Chip Hartranft, Gib and Faye Henderson, Claudia Ladensohn, and Mark Sorensen, for being friends in need, indeed.

Our friends give us wings and family gives us roots. My father, who passed away in 2006, accompanied me along the many twists and turns of my spiritual journey, including two trips to India together, until he couldn't anymore. My mother has been a staunch supporter of my interest in self-compassion since the beginning, generously trying out the self-compassion practices in her own life and sharing her experiences with me. That goes deep into the heart of a son. Gratitude also to my three rowdy brothers, who always thought the book should have been finished yesterday, and to my father's lovely second family, Maria, Anil, and Kamala.

I'd also like to offer each of my clients a deep bow because I can't thank them enough, or by name. They kept this project rooted in the reality of our daily lives as the words spilled onto the page, and gave it meaning and vitality.

The greatest debt is owed my wife, Claire. I'm acutely aware of the sacrifice a spouse makes to a book project. Besides feeling orphaned by a preoccupied partner, there are emotional ups and downs, an endless string of unexpected book-related tasks, and inevitable lost income. It's an act of faith to stay present in a relationship under these conditions. Claire has been the measure of balance that I often tried to convey throughout the book—somehow she knew just when to kiss and when to kick. Furthermore, she reviewed every line of the manuscript before I subjected my editors to it. We can still have epiphanies after decades of marriage—moments when we feel more loved than we love ourselves. Words cannot express my gratitude to Claire.

Going forward, I wish to humbly acknowledge the efforts of readers who will take the message of self-compassion to heart and make it live and breathe in their own lives. It's a path of peace and it's a blessing to share the journey together.

*   *   *

The following publishers and/or authors have generously given permission to reprint material from copyrighted works (in order of appearance in the book):

The Cartoon Bank, for "Jack and I ..." by Robert Weber (*cartoonbank.com*, 1994). Copyright 1994 by The New Yorker Collection. All rights reserved.

Beacon Press, for "Mindful" by Mary Oliver, from *Why I Wake Early* (Boston: Beacon Press, 2004). Copyright 2004 by Mary Oliver.

Black Sparrow Books, an imprint of David R. Godine, Publisher, for "Suddenly the City" by Linda Bamber, from *Metropolitan Tang* (Jaffrey, NH: Black Sparrow, 2008). Copyright 2008 by Linda Bamber.

The Cartoon Bank, for "Your own tedious thoughts ..." by Bruce Eric Kaplan (*cartoonbank.com,* 2002). Copyright 2002 by The New Yorker Collection. All rights reserved.

The Cartoon Bank, for "Lately I've been ..." by Lee Lorenz (*cartoonbank. com,* 1988). Copyright 1988 by The New Yorker Collection. All rights reserved.

Coleman Barks (trans.), for "The Guest House" by Rumi, from C. Barks and J. Moyne, *The Essential Rumi* (San Francisco: Harper, 1997). Originally published by Threshold Books. Copyright 1995 by Coleman Barks and John Moyne.

The Guilford Press, for an adaptation of "Table 1.1. Examples of Maladaptive Coping Responses" by Jeffrey E. Young, Janet S. Klosko, and Marjorie E. Weishaar, from *Schema Therapy: A Practitioner's Guide* (New York: Guilford Press, 2003). Copyright 2003 by The Guilford Press.

Farrar, Straus and Giroux, for "Love after Love" by Derek Walcott, from *Derek Walcott: Collected Poems, 1948–1984* (New York: Farrar, Straus and Giroux, 1987). Copyright 1986 by Derek Walcott.

Columbia University Press, for "I Can Wade Grief" by Emily Dickinson, from *The Columbia University Anthology of American Poetry* (New York: Columbia University Press, 1995).

Far Corner Books, for "Kindness" by Naomi Shihab Nye, from *Words under the Words: Selected Poems* (Portland, OR: Far Corner Books, 1995). Copyright 1995 by Naomi Shihab Nye.

New Directions Publishing Corp., for "When the Shoe Fits" by Thomas Merton, from *The Way of Chuang Tzu* (New York: New Directions, 1965). Copyright 1965 by the Abbey of Gethsemani.

The Cartoon Bank, for "Yeah, well, the Dalai Lama ..." by Bruce Eric Kaplan (*cartoonbank.com,* 2003). Copyright 2003 by The New Yorker Collection. All rights reserved.

David Sipress, for "May these people who cut in line ... ," from *Shambala Sun* (November 2007, p. 17). Copyright 2007 by David Sipress.

The Cartoon Bank, for "Are we there yet?" by David Sipress (*cartoonbank. com,* 1998). Copyright 1998 by The New Yorker Collection. All rights reserved.

Steven J. DeRose, for "The Compass DeRose Guide to Emotion Words," by Steven J. DeRose (*www.derose.net/steve/resources/emotionwords/ewords.html,* July 6, 2005). Copyright 2005 by Steven J. DeRose.

introduction

Life is tough. Despite our best intentions, things go wrong, sometimes *very* wrong. Ninety percent of us get married, full of hope and optimism, yet 40% of marriages end in divorce. We struggle to meet the demands of daily life, only to find ourselves needing care for stress-related problems like high blood pressure, anxiety, depression, alcoholism, or a weakened immune system.

How do we typically react when things fall apart? More often than not, we feel ashamed and become self-critical: "What's wrong with me?" "Why can't I cope?" "Why me?" Perhaps we go on a mission to fix ourselves, adding insult to injury. Sometimes we go after others. Rather than giving ourselves a break, we seem to find the path of greatest resistance.

Yet no matter how hard we try to avoid emotional pain, it follows us everywhere. Difficult emotions—shame, anger, loneliness, fear, despair, confusion—arrive like clockwork at our door. They come when things don't go according to our expectations, when we're separated from loved ones, and as a part of ordinary sickness, old age, and death. It's just not possible to avoid feeling bad.

But we *can* learn to deal with misery and distress in a new, healthier way. Instead of greeting difficult emotions by fighting hard against them, we can *bear witness to our own pain and respond with kind-*

1

ness and understanding. That's self-compassion—taking care of ourselves just as we'd treat someone we love dearly. If you're used to beating yourself up during periods of sadness or loneliness, if you hide from the world when you make a mistake, or if you obsess over how you could have prevented the mistake to begin with, self-compassion may seem like a radical idea. But why should you deny yourself the same tenderness and warmth you extend to others who are suffering?

When we fight emotional pain, we get trapped in it. Difficult emotions become *destructive* and break down the mind, body, and spirit. Feelings get stuck—frozen in time—and we get stuck in them. The happiness we long for in relationships seems to elude us. Satisfaction at work lies just beyond our reach. We drag ourselves through the day, arguing with our physical aches and pains. Usually we're not aware just how many of these trials have their root in how we *relate* to the inevitable discomfort of life.

Change comes naturally when we open ourselves to emotional pain with uncommon kindness. Instead of blaming, criticizing, and trying to fix ourselves (or someone else, or the whole world) when things go wrong and we feel bad, we can start with self-acceptance. Compassion first! This simple shift can make a tremendous difference in your life.

Imagine that your partner just criticized you for yelling at your daughter. This hurts your feelings and leads to an argument. Perhaps you felt misunderstood, disrespected, unloved, or unlovable? Maybe you didn't use the right words to describe how you felt, but more likely your partner was being too angry or defensive to hear what you had to say. Now imagine that you took a deep breath and said the following to yourself *before* the argument: "More than anything, I want to be a good parent. It's so painful to me when I yell at my child. I love my daughter more than anything in the world, but sometimes I just lose it. I'm only human, I guess. May I learn to forgive myself for my mistakes, and may we find a way to live together in peace." Can you feel the difference?

A moment of self-compassion like this can change your entire day. A string of such moments can change the course of your life.

Freeing yourself from the trap of destructive thoughts and emotions through self-compassion can boost your self-esteem from the inside out, reduce depression and anxiety, and even help you stick to your diet.

And the benefits aren't just personal. Self-compassion is the foundation of compassion for others. The Dalai Lama said, "[Compassion] is the state of wishing that the object of our compassion be free of suffering. ... Yourself first, and then in a more advanced way the aspiration will embrace others." It makes sense, doesn't it, that we won't be able to empathize with others if we can't tolerate the same feelings—despair, fear, failure, shame—occurring within ourselves? And how can we pay the slightest attention to others when we're absorbed in our own internal struggles? When our problems become workable again, we can extend kindness to others, which can only help improve relationships and enhance our overall contentment and satisfaction with life.

Self-compassion is really the most natural thing in the world. Think about it for a minute. If you cut your finger, you'll want to clean it, bandage it, and help it heal. That's innate self-compassion. But where does self-compassion go when our *emotional* well-being is at stake? What's effective for survival against a saber-tooth tiger doesn't seem to work in emotional life. We instinctively go to battle against unpleasant emotions as if they were external foes, and fighting them inside only makes matters worse. Resist anxiety and it can turn into full-blown panic. Suppress grief and chronic depression may develop. Struggling to fall asleep can keep you awake all night long.

When we're caught up in our pain, we also go to war against *ourselves.* The body protects itself against danger through fight, flight, or freeze (staying frozen in place), but when we're challenged emotionally, these reactions become an unholy trinity of self-criticism, self-isolation, and self-absorption. A healing alternative is to cultivate a new relationship to ourselves described by research psychologist Kristin Neff as self-kindness, a sense of connection with the rest of humanity, and balanced awareness. That's self-compassion.

In this book you'll discover how to bring self-compassion to your emotional life when you need it most—when you're dying of shame, when you grind your teeth in rage or fear, or when you're too fragile to face yet another family gathering. Self-compassion is giving yourself the love you need by boosting your innate wish to be happy and free from suffering.

Dealing with emotional pain without making it worse is the essence of Buddhist psychology. The ideas in this book draw from that tradition, particularly those concepts and practices that have been validated by modern science. What you'll read is essentially old wine in new bottles—ancient insights in modern psychological idiom. You don't have to believe in anything to make the practices work for you—you can be a Christian, a Jew, a Muslim, a scientist, or a skeptic. The best approach is to be open-minded, experimental, and flexible.

Clinical scientists discovered meditation in the 1970s, and it's now one of the most thoroughly researched of all psychotherapy methods. Over the past 15 years, research has focused primarily on *mindfulness*, or "awareness of present experience, with acceptance." Mindfulness is considered an underlying factor in effective psycho-therapy and emotional healing in general. When therapy goes well, patients (or clients) develop an accepting attitude toward whatever they're experiencing in the therapy room—fear, anger, sadness, joy, relief, boredom, love—and this benevolent attitude gets transferred to daily life. A special bonus of mindfulness is that it can be prac-ticed at home in the form of meditation.

Mindfulness tends to focus on the *experience* of a person, usually a sensation, thought, or feeling. But what do we do when the *expe-riencer* is overcome with emotion, perhaps with shame or self-doubt? When that happens, we don't just *feel* bad—we feel we *are* bad. We can become so rattled that it's hard to pay attention to anything at all. What do we do when we're alone in the middle of the night, twisting the sheets around us in bed, sleep medication isn't working, and therapy is a week away? Mostly we need a good friend with a compassionate heart. If one isn't immediately available, we can still give kindness to ourselves—self-compassion.

I encountered self-compassion from two directions, one professional and one personal. I've practiced psychotherapy for 30 years with patients ranging from the worried well to those overwhelmed by anxiety, depression, or trauma. I also worked in a public hospital with people suffering from chronic and terminal illnesses. Over the years, I've witnessed the power of compassion, how it opens the heart like a flower, revealing and healing hidden sorrow. After therapy, however, some patients feel like they're walking into a void with the voice of the therapist trailing far behind. I wondered, "What can people do *between* sessions to feel less vulnerable and alone?" Sometimes I asked myself, "Is there any way to make the therapy experience rub off more quickly—to make it *portable*?" Self-compassion seems to hold that promise for many people.

Personally, I was raised by a devout Christian mother and a father who spent 9 years in India during early adulthood, mostly interned by the British during World War II because he was a German citizen. There my father met a mountaineer, Heinrich Harrer, who later escaped the internment camp and traveled across the Himalayan mountains to Tibet to became the 14th Dalai Lama's English tutor. As a child, my mother read me magical tales of India, so it seemed natural to go there myself after I graduated from college. From 1976 to 1977, I traveled the length and breadth of India, visiting saints, sages, and shamans, and I learned Buddhist meditation in a cave in Sri Lanka. Thus began a lifelong interest in meditation and over a dozen return trips to India.

I currently practice meditation in the insight meditation tradition found in the American centers established by Sharon Salzberg, Joseph Goldstein, and Jack Kornfield. Those rich and nuanced teachings inform this entire book, and any unwarranted deviation from them is my responsibility alone. I also owe an immeasurable debt of gratitude to my colleagues at the Institute for Meditation and Psychotherapy, with whom I've been in monthly conversation for almost 25 years, and to Jon Kabat-Zinn, who introduced the Buddhist practice of mindfulness and compassion into modern health care. My other teachers are my patients, who have generously offered their life stories to give substance to the concepts and practices that follow. They made this a labor of love. Their names and other details have been changed to ensure confidentiality, and some clinical vignettes are composites of a few individuals.

This book is divided into three parts, and the chapters build on one another. Part I, Discovering Self-Compassion, shows you how to develop mindfulness and describes precisely what we mean and don't mean by self-compassion. Part II, Practicing Loving-Kindness, gives in-depth instruction in one particular self-compassion practice—loving-kindness meditation—to serve as a foundation for a compassionate way of life. Part III, Customizing Self-Compassion, offers tips for adjusting the practice to your particular personality and circumstances and shows you how to achieve maximum benefit from the practice. Finally, in the appendices, you'll find additional self-compassion exercises and resources for further reading and more intensive practice.

This book will not be a lot of work. The hard work is actually behind you—fighting and resisting difficult feelings, blaming yourself for them and their causes. You'll actually learn to work *less*. It's an "un-self-help book." Instead of beginning with the notion that something about you is broken and needs to be fixed, I hope to show you how to respond to emotional pain in a new, more compassionate, and loving way. I recommend you try the exercises for 30 days and see how it goes. You might notice yourself feeling lighter and happier, but that will simply be a by-product of accepting yourself just as you are.

Part I

discovering
self–compassion

1

being kind to yourself

The suffering itself is not so bad; it's the resentment against suffering that is the real pain.
—ALLEN GINSBERG, *poet*

"I'm afraid of what you're about to tell me, 'cause it probably won't work!" Michelle blurted out, fully expecting to be disappointed by what I had to say. Michelle had just finished telling me about her years of struggle with shyness, and I was taking a deep breath.

Michelle struck me as an exceptionally bright and conscientious person. She had read many books on overcoming shyness and tried therapy four times. She didn't want to be let down again. She'd recently received an MBA from a prestigious university and gotten a job as a consultant to large firms in the area. The main problem for Michelle was blushing. She believed it signaled to others that she wasn't competent and that they shouldn't trust what she had to say. The more she worried about blushing, the more she actually blushed in front of others. Her new job was an important career opportunity, and Michelle didn't want to blow it.

I assured Michelle that she was right: whatever I suggested *wouldn't* work. That's not because she was a lost cause—far from it—but rather because all well-intentioned strategies are destined to fail. It's not the fault of the techniques, nor is it the fault of the person who wants to feel better. The problem lies in our motivation and in a misunderstanding of how the mind works.

As Michelle knew only too well from her years of struggle, a lot of what we do to *not* feel bad is likely to make us feel worse. It's like that thought experiment: "Try not to think about pink elephants—the kind that are *very* large and *very* pink." Once an idea is planted in our minds, it's strengthened every time we try not to think about it. Sigmund Freud summed up the problem by saying there's "no negation" in the unconscious mind. Similarly, whatever we throw at our distress to make it go away—relaxation techniques, blocking our thoughts, positive affirmations—will ultimately disappoint, and we'll have no choice but to set off to find another option to feel better.

While we were discussing these matters, Michelle began to weep gently. I wasn't sure whether she was feeling *more* disheartened or in some way the truth of her experience was being articulated. She told me that even her prayers were going unanswered. We talked about two types of prayers: the kind where we want God to make bad things go away and the kind where we surrender—"Let go and let God." Michelle said it had never occurred to her to surrender her troubles to God. That wasn't her style.

Gradually we came around to what could be done for Michelle that might actually decrease her anxiety and blushing—not deep breathing, not pinching herself, not drinking cold water, not pretending to be unflappable. Since Michelle wasn't the kind of person to relax her efforts, she needed to find something entirely different. Michelle recognized that her anxiety decreased the *more* she accepted it, and it *increased* the *less* she accepted it. Hence, it made sense to Michelle to dedicate herself to a life of *accepting* anxiety and the fact that she was simply an anxious person. Our therapy was to be measured not by how often she blushed, but by how accepting she was of her blushing. That was a radical new idea for Michelle. She left our first session elated, if a bit perplexed.

She sent me an e-mail during the following week, happily announcing that "it worked." Since we hadn't discussed any new practices, I wasn't sure what Michelle meant. Later I learned that she had begun saying to herself "just scared, just scared" whenever she noticed she was anxious. Labeling her fear seemed to take Michelle's mind off how flushed her face felt, and she was able to chat briefly with colleagues in the lunchroom without incident, for example. She was relieved to feel more like "a scared person getting lunch" than like a "weak, overly sensitive, ridiculous person who didn't know what she was talking about." I marveled at how Michelle had taken the concept of "acceptance" and invented a useful technique in such a short time.

At our next meeting, however, Michelle was discouraged again. Her forays into the lunchroom once again became a battle against the blush. Her original wish to "stop looking anxious" reasserted itself. Acceptance had begun to "work" for Michelle, but she'd let go of her newfound commitment to cultivate acceptance. She mistakenly believed she'd found a clever bypass to her problem.

Unfortunately, we can't trick ourselves. There was a part of Michelle that was saying, "I'm practicing acceptance *in order to* reduce anxiety." But that's not acceptance. Within modern psychology, *acceptance* means to embrace whatever arises within us, moment to moment, just as it is. Sometimes it's a feeling we like; sometimes it's a bad feeling. We naturally want to continue the good feelings and stop the bad ones, but setting out with that goal doesn't work. The only answer to our problems is to first *have* our problems, fully and completely, whatever they may be. Michelle was hoping to skip that part.

This story has a happy ending, which was reached slowly over the course of 2 years. Michelle discovered how to live in accord with her sensitive nervous system. Relapses reliably occurred when Michelle tried *not* to blush, but she hardly blushed at all when she was ready to let blushing take its course. As Michelle made her peace with blushing, she found she could apply the same principles to other stress symptoms that inevitably arose during her day—tension in her chest, headaches, heart palpitations—and her life became much easier.

This is a book about how we can benefit by *turning toward our emotional pain*. That's a tall order. Any thinking person is likely to ask, "Why would I want to do *that*?" In this chapter, you'll see why it's often the best thing to do. The rest of the book will show you how to accomplish this improbable task. First you'll learn how to bring mindful awareness to what's bothering you. Then you'll discover how to bring kindness to *yourself,* especially when you're feeling really bad. That combination—mindfulness and self-compassion— can transform even the worst times of our lives.

TURNING TOWARD THE PAIN

From the moment of our birth, we're on a quest for happiness. It may take no more than mother's milk to satisfy us in the first days of our lives, but our needs and desires multiply as we age. By adulthood, most of us don't expect to be happy unless we have a nice family, a good job, excellent health, lots of money, and the love and admiration of others.

But pain still strikes even under the best of circumstances. Billionaire Howard Hughes found himself desperate and alone at the moment of his death. And our circumstances inevitably change; one person's marriage may fall apart, another may have a child with a developmental disability, and yet another may lose everything in a flood. People differ from one another in the *amount* of suffering they endure over a lifetime, or in the *type* of suffering, but none of us gets off without any. Pain and suffering are common threads that unite all of humanity.

Pain creates a conflict between the way things are and how we'd like them to be and that makes our lives feel *unsatisfactory*. The more we wish our lives were different, the worse we feel. For example, if a car accident lands someone in a wheelchair for life, the first year is usually the toughest. As we learn to adapt, we typically return to our former level of happiness. We can measure our happiness by the gap between what we want and how things are.

The Hedonic Treadmill

In 1971, Philip Brickman and Donald Campbell proposed that we're on a pleasure-seeking treadmill, vainly trying to achieve happiness by seeking what's just around the corner—a better relationship, an easier job, a nicer car. The problem is that our nervous systems quickly adapt to anything familiar. Once you get a nice new car, how long do you enjoy it before thinking about renovating your home? Studies show that most lottery winners are ultimately no happier than nonwinners, and paraplegics usually become as content as people who can walk. For better or worse, we adapt to both good and bad life events. This general adaptation theory has held up empirically for decades, with some recent modifications that you will read about in Chapter 5.

When we're on the hedonic treadmill for too long, though, it can lead to exhaustion and disease. In his immensely entertaining and informative book on the causes and consequences of stress, *Why Zebras Don't Get Ulcers*, Robert Sapolsky describes how animals are perfectly adapted to respond to physical crises. Consider a zebra running from a lion that wants to rip out its stomach; when the danger passes, the zebra goes back to grazing peacefully. But what do humans do? We anticipate danger lurking around the corner. Sapolsky asks, "How many hippos worry about whether Social Security is going to last as long as they will, or what they are going to say on a first date?" Our bodies react to *psychological* threats the same way they react to physical threats, and a sense of constant danger raises our overall stress level and the risk of heart disease, immune dysfunction, depression, colitis, chronic pain, memory impairment, sexual problems, and much more.

The exact mechanism by which psychological stress leads to disease is unclear, but preliminary evidence shows that it may be related to your telomeres—DNA-protein complexes at the ends of chromosomes. Cells age—they stop dividing—when they lose their telomeric DNA. Life stress has been shown to shorten the telomeres in the immune system, and fewer immune cells can lead to disease and shorten your lifespan.

Most of us believe that our happiness depends on the *external* circumstances of our lives. Therefore, we spend our lives on a treadmill, continually arranging to have pleasure and avoid pain. When we experience pleasure, we *grasp* for more of it. When we experience pain, we *avoid* it. Both of these reactions are instinctive, but they're not successful strategies for emotional well-being. The problem with pleasure seeking is that the pleasure will end at some point and we'll become disappointed: we fall out of love, our bellies become full, our friends go home. The problem with avoiding pain is that it's just not possible to do, and it often gets worse with our increased efforts to try. For example, eating to reduce stress can cause obesity, and working excessively to overcome low self-esteem can land you in the grave.

It's possible to be completely controlled by the instinct to seek pleasure and avoid pain. I know a man, Stewart, who took great pleasure in drinking alcohol when he was younger. He started drinking when he was 14 years old. By the time Stewart was 20, he routinely drank a case of beer (24 cans) per night. One evening he had a panic attack while he was drunk, and it so frightened him that he never drank again. Beer, the source of so much pleasure, had become terrifying overnight because he associated it with his panic attack. Stewart then stopped going anywhere or doing anything that could possibly trigger a panic attack, including other things he used to enjoy, such as driving his truck around town and going to baseball games. First the pleasure of alcohol dominated his life, then the fear of a panic attack did. Stewart was a hostage to these short-term states of mind: pleasure and pain.

A new approach is to change our *relationship* to pain and pleasure. We can step back and learn to be calm in the midst of pain; we can let pleasure naturally come and go. That's serenity. We can even learn to *embrace* pain as well as pleasure, and every nuance in between, thereby living each moment to the fullest. That's joy. Learning how to spend some time with pain is essential to achieving personal happiness. It may sound paradoxical, but in order to be happy we must embrace *un*happiness.

Embracing Misery in Marriage

For 14 years, psychologist John Gottman and colleagues at the University of Washington tracked 650 couples to discover what made marriages successful. He says he's able to predict with 91% accuracy which couples will end up in divorce. They're the ones who practice criticism, defensiveness, contempt, and stonewalling, the "Four Horsemen of the Apocalypse." Gottman also observed that 69% of marital disputes are never resolved, especially arguments about core personality issues and values. Since couples don't resolve most of their personal differences, successful couples somehow learn to accept them. Happy couples "know each other intimately and they are well versed in each other's likes, dislikes, personality quirks, hopes and dreams."

Psychologists Andrew Christensen and Neil Jacobson developed an acceptance-based couple therapy: integrative couple therapy. This approach uses behavior therapy to address problems that *can* be changed and "acceptance" for problems that can't change. Acceptance means embracing problems as a path to intimacy and relinquishing the need to change one's partner. In a randomized, controlled study of 6 months of weekly couple therapy, two-thirds of couples that were chronically distressed before treatment remained significantly improved 2 years later.

WHAT WE RESIST PERSISTS

There's a simple formula that captures our instinctive response to pain:

$$\text{Pain} \times \text{Resistance} = \text{Suffering}$$

"Pain" refers to unavoidable discomfort that comes into our lives, such as an accident, an illness, or the death of someone we love. "Resistance" refers to any effort to ward off pain, such as tensing the body or ruminating about how to make pain go away. "Suffering" is what results when we resist pain. Suffering is the physical and emotional tension that we *add* to our pain, layer upon layer.

In this formula, how we relate to pain determines how much we'll suffer. As our resistance to pain is reduced to zero, so is our suffering. Pain times zero equals zero. Hard to believe? The pain of life is there, but we don't unnecessarily elaborate on it. We don't carry it with us everywhere we go.

An example of suffering is spending hours and hours thinking about how we should have sold our stocks before the market collapsed or worrying that we might get sick before a big upcoming event. Some amount of reflection is necessary to anticipate and prevent problems, but we often get stuck regretting the past or worrying about the future.

Pain is inevitable; suffering is optional. It seems that the more intense our emotional pain is, the more we suffer by obsessing, blaming ourselves, and feeling defective. The good news is that since most of the pain in our lives is really suffering—the result of fighting

The Benefit of Worry

Why can't we seem to stop worrying? Tom Borkovec at the Pennsylvania State University asked 45 students who were afraid of public speaking to imagine a scary scene 10 times. "Imagine you are about to present an important speech to a large audience. ... As you stand there, you can feel your heart pounding fast ..." Before doing that, Borkovec had three different groups engage in relaxed, neutral, or worrisome thinking. Then, while they imagined the scary scene, he measured the students' heart rate. Surprisingly, the group of students who were instructed to worry beforehand had *no increase in heart rate* compared to those who didn't. This means that worrying actually stopped the body from being aroused by fear, which unconsciously encourages us to worry more. Unfortunately, those participants who worried in advance actually *felt more afraid* while actively visualizing a scary situation, even though the heart rate didn't increase.

the experience of pain—we can actually *do* something about it. Let's take a look at four common problems—lower back pain, insomnia, anxiety about public speaking, and relational conflict—and start to consider how they can be alleviated by acceptance and letting go.

Chronic Back Pain

Chronic back pain is a debilitating ailment. Unfortunately, it's very common in the United States, affecting at least five million people at any given time: 60–70% of Americans get lower back pain sometime in their lives. Surprisingly, two-thirds of people *without* chronic back pain have the same structural back problems as those who experience pain. So what's going on in the bodies and minds of those suffering from chronic pain? Resistance. Let's consider the case of Mira.

Mira is a 49-year-old yoga enthusiast with a successful business career. She is not the kind of person you'd expect to have back pain, except that she pursues all her activities with uncommon zeal. During a particularly strenuous yoga session, Mira felt a twinge while doing a forward bend. She then felt her sciatic nerve tingle right down to her calves. Almost any position except standing straight up or lying flat gave her back pain. An MRI (magnetic resonance imaging) diagnosed her with a herniated disk, a painful condition where the bones of the spine squeeze the disk out against a nerve.

Mira stopped doing yoga and saw a physical therapist who taught her to lift objects in such a way that her back stayed straight and didn't give her any pain. But over time, her back hurt more and more. She was also deeply unhappy that she couldn't exercise vigorously, her primary way of relieving work stress. She envisioned a lifetime without mountain climbing, bicycle riding, or yoga. Mira also blamed herself for causing her disk to herniate in the first place. The combination of worry, self-criticism, mounting tension from inactivity, and increasing back pain convinced Mira to turn to surgery.

Prior to her operation, Mira did some research and learned that the long-term success rate of back surgery for herniated disks was no better than having no surgery at all. She also read Ronald Siegel's book *Back Sense,* which explains that for most sufferers the most valuable treatment for a herniated disk is to reduce anxiety about the pain and resume normal activities as soon as possible. That meant lifting objects in roughly the same manner as always so that the back muscles don't atrophy from inactivity. Mira found out that persistent muscle tension, not structural abnormalities, causes most chronic back pain. And muscle tension increases both when the muscles are not used and when we worry. On top of this, worry amplifies pain signals, further adding to our experience of pain.

Mira took these messages to heart. She got massage therapy for her sore muscles, used a heating pad every evening, and began exercising in moderation. Her anxiety decreased as her pain subsided, and her back pain diminished by 50% in less than 2 weeks.

Most people who suffer from chronic back pain will say that Mira was just lucky, an exception. Actually, she's the rule. Ironically the prevalence of chronic back pain is lowest in developing countries, where people do *more* backbreaking work than in industrialized countries. An injury is usually the trigger for a back problem, but injury isn't what *sustained* Mira's back pain. Her resistance to the pain, especially fearing that she wouldn't be able to continue her vigorous lifestyle, pulled Mira deeper and deeper down into

Job Dissatisfaction Predicts Chronic Low Back Pain

Low back pain is one of the most common and costly reasons for workplace disability. Psychosocial factors seem to predict disability more than physical problems. In a study by Rebecca Williams and colleagues, 82 men between 18 and 52 years old with back pain for 6 to 10 weeks were assessed to see if job satisfaction predicts pain, psychological distress, and/or disability. Six months later, workers who were *satisfied* with their jobs had less pain and disability from back pain, and there was a tendency toward less psychological distress. Social status and the type of work did not affect the results of this study. These findings suggest that when employment is a source of satisfaction, people are likely to continue working *despite* low back pain. They resume normal behavior.

her health crisis. Acceptance of physical pain, and working *with* it, returned Mira to her normal life.

Insomnia

Most of us have suffered from insomnia at some point in our lives. Up to half of the adult population in the United States reports having insomnia in any given year. The physical causes are numerous and include trying to sleep beside a snoring partner, consuming caffeine before bedtime, napping too often, exercising too little, taking medications like cold tablets, and having sleep apnea. Regardless of the causes, many of us find we make matters worse by trying too hard to fall asleep. How does this happen?

Try to remember the last time you had an important meeting scheduled early the next morning and you found yourself lying awake late into the night. Perhaps it was a job interview, or perhaps you had to make a presentation at work. As you lay there, you couldn't stop thinking that every hour of wakefulness would be translated into a more distracted and sluggish mind. You became increasingly annoyed with yourself with each passing hour, perhaps concluding that you had entirely lost the ability to sleep normally. And every time you looked at the clock, you felt an annoying surge of adrenaline in your chest or the pit of your stomach.

The source of this problem is that the nervous system moves into "fight-or-flight" mode when you battle to fall asleep. It's a vicious cycle: trying to sleep stresses the body into wakefulness. We need to break the cycle by abandoning the fight. There are a number of ways that people try to accomplish this:

1. Remember how well you actually function on less sleep; most people do. This may soften the feeling of urgency.

2. Notice that lying peacefully in bed is a form of valuable rest in itself, whether or not you fall asleep.

3. Remember that the body will demand sleep when it really needs it, which isn't in this moment.

4. Dedicate 30 minutes to being fully awake, which might be enough time for the mind to shut off and begin to sleep.

5. Reinforce your intention to accept sleeplessness by emphatically saying "I don't care!" whenever you discover that you're still awake.

6. Count your breaths.

However, as any insomniac will tell you, even these tricks don't work much of the time. Why? Because you can't fool the mind—it knows that you're doing these things to fall asleep. There's a big difference, for example, between "counting your breaths" and "counting your breaths *to fall asleep.*" At a subtle level, when your agenda is to fall asleep, you can't help getting upset with yourself when you realize you're still awake. Every passing hour makes you feel more desperate and confused. To solve the problem, your *relationship* to sleeplessness has to shift. Once you begin to truly, genuinely *accept* not sleeping, your body will finally get a chance to rest.

Fear of Public Speaking

Jerry Seinfeld quipped, "According to most studies, people's number-one fear is public speaking. Number two is death. Death is number two. Does that sound right? This means to the average person, if you go to a funeral, you're better off in the casket than doing the eulogy."

Fear of public speaking is indeed very common—at least a third of us feel that our anxiety is "excessive" when we're in front of an audience. One out of 10 people find it has interfered markedly in their work. I've also struggled with public-speaking anxiety. Here's what happens to me.

If I have an important speech scheduled, I can feel tension in my abdomen—a little surge of adrenaline, a little muscular contraction—whenever I think about it. This predictable annoyance happens especially when I'm planning to speak on a new topic and I haven't prepared what I'm going to say yet. I imagine myself clearing my

Suppress It!

The young Dostoyevsky is said to have challenged his brother to *not* think of a white bear, leaving him puzzled and confused. In 1987, Daniel Wegner and colleagues asked students to do the same thought suppression task for 5 minutes, ringing a bell each time they thought of a white bear as they simultaneously verbalized whatever came to their minds. Thereafter, this group was asked to *intentionally* think of a white bear and perform the same tasks. (A comparison group was asked to think of a white bear for the entire 10 minutes.) Not only was the first group, the suppression group, unable to suppress the thought of white bears during the first 5 minutes, but this group also thought of white bears even *more* during the second 5-minute period than the group that never suppressed. This classic study shows that suppression creates the very preoccupation that it's directed against. Clinical researchers speculate that a similar process may underlie psychological disorders such as posttraumatic stress, depression, and obsessive–compulsive disorder—the thoughts we push away come back to haunt us.

In another study, this time on *emotional* suppression, researchers at Florida State University asked students not to cringe while watching a slaughterhouse movie and not to laugh during a Jay Leno comedy clip. They were then asked to complete a difficult finger-tracing task. The attempt to control emotional reactions to the films made blood glucose levels decrease, and students with lower glucose levels gave up earlier on the finger-tracing task. When the same participants were given sugary drinks to reverse glucose depletion, they persisted longer with the task. Emotional suppression seems to reduce will-power, and lowered glucose may be one reason for it.

These two studies help to explain why trying to resist a chocolate cookie is such a difficult, and often unsuccessful, task.

throat too many times, fumbling for words, making jokes no one laughs at, and watching the audience's distress on my behalf. Maybe someone in the audience, trying to be helpful, yells out something like "Take a breath!" (That scenario actually happened to me.)

Behind my fear is the desire to be liked: to appear intelligent and charming and not to bore the audience. I have the false notion that if everyone in the audience approved of me, I'd be truly content. But there's another reason to give public speeches: to communicate something of value to others. One strategy I've used to overcome public-speaking anxiety is to reorient myself toward the actual message I wish to deliver. For example, if the subject is brain science, I'll commit myself to delivering a few useful points about brain science before the speech is over. Taking the focus away from "me" seems to help.

Regrettably, this technique is only a partial solution if I harbor an underlying wish not to look nervous in front of an audience. Joseph Goldstein, a meditation teacher, says "Life occurs at the tip of motivation." What am I trying to achieve while speaking? Not looking nervous? If so, there will be a small monitor in my head that asks, "Are you nervous? ... Are you nervous *now*?" That nagging question evokes the very anxiety I'm trying to suppress, and once I'm anxious I become anxious about being anxious.

The only lasting solution to public-speaking anxiety is simply to be anxious. We must stop shielding ourselves from anxiety—be willing to tremble and speak at the same time. My anxiety doesn't last very long if I do that. Even far in advance of a public talk, my willingness to be anxious stops the whole negative feedback loop.

Relationship Conflict

Relationships go through good times and bad as the tide of connection ebbs and flows. If we want a feeling of connection—feeling seen and heard, resonating, "on the same page"—and it isn't forthcoming, we feel pain. All couples have painful periods, sometimes for extended periods of time:

Suzanne and Michael were going through "cold hell." Cold hell is a state in which couples feel resentful and suspicious of each other and communicate in chilly, carefully modulated tones. Some couples can go on like this for years, frozen on the brink of divorce.

After 5 months of unsuccessful therapy, meeting every other

week, Suzanne decided it was time to file for divorce. It seemed obvious to her that Michael would never change—that he would not work less than 65 hours a week or take care of himself (he was 50 pounds overweight and smoked). Even more distressing to Suzanne was the fact that Michael was making no effort to enjoy their marriage; they seldom went out and had not taken a vacation in 2½ years. Suzanne felt lonely and rejected. Michael felt unappreciated for working so hard to take care of his family.

Suzanne's move toward divorce was the turning point—it gave them "the gift of desperation." For the first time, Michael seemed willing to explore just how painful his life had become. During one session, when they were discussing a heavy snowstorm in the Denver area, Michael mentioned that his 64-year-old father had just missed his first day of work in 20 years. I asked Michael what that meant to him. His eyes welling up with tears, Michael said he wished his father had enjoyed his life more. I wondered aloud if Michael had ever wished the same thing for himself. "I'm scared," he replied. "I'm scared of what would happen if I stopped working all the time. I'm even scared to stop worrying about the business—scared that I might be overlooking something important that would make my whole business crumble before my eyes."

With that, a light went on for Suzanne. "Is that why you ignore me and the kids and even ignore your own body?" she asked him. Michael just nodded, his tears flowing freely now. "Oh my God," Suzanne said. "I thought it was me—that I wasn't good enough, that I'm just too much trouble for you. We're both anxious—just in different ways. You're scared about your business and I'm scared about our marriage. I live in fear of our marriage crumbling *every single day* while you're at work." The frozen feeling of disconnection that had separated Michael and Suzanne for years had begun to thaw.

From the beginning of our sessions, Michael had been aware of his workaholism. He even realized that he was ignoring his family just as he had been ignored by his own father. But Michael felt helpless to reverse the intergenerational transmission of suffering. That began to change when he felt the pain of the impending divorce. Michael accepted how unhappy his life had become, and he expe-

rienced a spark of compassion, first for his father and then for himself.

Suzanne often complained that Michael paid insufficient attention to their two kids. But behind her complaints was a wish—not
unfamiliar to mothers of young children—that Michael would pay
attention to her first when he came home from work, and later play
with the kids. Suzanne was ashamed of this desire; she thought it
was selfish and indicated that she was a bad mother. But when she
could see it as a natural expression of her wish to connect with her
husband, she was able to make her request more openly and confi-
dently. Michael, in turn, found it much easier to respond to these
requests.

A little self-acceptance and self-compassion allowed both
Suzanne and Michael to begin to transform their difficult emotions.
In relationships, behind strong feelings like shame and anger is often
a big "I MISS YOU!" It simply feels unnatural and painful not to
feel connected with our loved ones.

Despite the obvious differences between public-speaking anxiety, back pain, insomnia, and relational conflict, they usually share
a common ingredient: resistance to discomfort. Fighting what we're
uneasy about only makes things worse. The more we can accept
the anxiety, physical discomfort, sleeplessness, and pain of disconnection—and the self-doubt that goes along with it—the better off
we'll be.

You can surely recognize the same dynamic in your own life.
How successful is your diet if you're overly strict and self-critical
about it? What happens when you argue with your teenage daughter
about her new boyfriend? Where does your anger go when you suppress it? A colleague of mine quipped, "When you resist something,
it goes to the basement and lifts weights!"

At the severe end of the spectrum, trying not to feel ashamed
by attacking others, verbally or physically, can destroy relationships
and even lives. Drinking to reduce anxiety or block out traumatic
memories can take away everything you have or ever wanted to
have. Cutting one's own skin to get relief from emotional pain

solves nothing. The challenge is to turn toward our difficulties with nonjudgmental awareness and compassion. This book was written to start you down that more fruitful path.

FINDING THE MIDDLE WAY

It's asking a lot to open yourself to discomfort. When I made the decision to allow myself to tremble in front of an audience, I had to think through what that actually meant. Not just *think* about it, actually *shudder* through the scene: people laughing at me, telling one another about my poor performance, turning away in embarrassed dismay. Only then could I see that my life would go on if I were a dud as a speaker. It was a kind of exposure therapy—getting used to it in my imagination; fortunately or unfortunately, I had some actual experience to go on.

Some people can simply jump in and embrace their emotional distress. Others take a more gradual path. Hurling themselves into those turbulent waters works for some people, but the willingness to do so is no indication of personal virtue—especially if you can't swim. You must feel safe and competent before taking that first step toward pain.

Most of us worry about what could happen if we opened up to emotional pain. Depressed people may fear they'll be overwhelmed and unable to function. Those with anxiety worry that it will set them back, giving them yet another vivid instance of anxiety to remember. People with a trauma background expect scary memories to break through and haunt them during the day. Those in difficult marriages may worry that they'll have to take action on their relationships if they allow themselves to feel how bad things have become. These are all real possibilities for which we should be prepared.

The purpose of this book is to teach you the knowledge and the skills to face suffering from a position of strength. What this book cannot teach is *intuition* about whether it's safe for you, at any particular moment, to turn toward pain. You have to decide that for yourself. We're all sensitive beings, even if we don't show it. We have fragile nervous systems. Learn to use your intuition to distinguish between "safety" and "discomfort." Feeling vulnerable or uncomfortable doesn't necessarily mean you're unsafe; "hurt" does not necessarily mean "harm." It's important to know the difference if you want to live your life to its fullest.

We usually tolerate all manner of difficulties to lead a meaningful life. For example, if having children is important to you, you'll probably risk the pain of childbirth to pursue your dream. Wisdom is the quality of knowing the short- and long-term consequences of our actions and choosing the path of greatest long-term benefit. Sticking to our deepest commitments and values, despite the obstacles, is wise because it yields long-term happiness.

It's best to seek a "middle way" between facing and avoiding your difficulties. You might feel fragile one day and unable to meet your challenges. If so, perhaps they can wait. Imagine you're on a ski vacation. Some days you may want to attempt double-diamond slopes, and other days you may just want to sip hot chocolate in the lodge. If you try a steep slope when you're not prepared, you may crash. If you stick to the bunny slopes, you won't enjoy the thrill of mastery. Given the choice, attempt new challenges only when you're good and ready. But don't give up either.

Some people wonder how antidepressant and anti-anxiety medications fit into this picture. Aren't they just forms of avoidance, delaying or burying emotional challenges? That may be so in some cases, but generally speaking our problems are unworkable when we're overwhelmed with fear, sadness, or disorganized thinking. Avoidance is good if it helps us regain perspective. Medication can bring emotional suffering down to a manageable level. Some people may eventually be able to reduce their medication using self-regulation strategies such as those described in this book.

The mind has its own natural ways of avoiding distress. These are our "defense mechanisms," such as "denial," "projection," and "splitting." Splitting, for example, refers to the mind's tendency to see things as black or white when we're under threat: "He's all good;

she's all bad." It comforts us to think that way. *Denial* is the refusal to accept something that causes anxiety, such as a partner being an alcoholic or having an affair. *Projection* is when we shift our unacceptable feelings and impulses onto another person to feel better about ourselves, such as "He's a racist" or "She's just jealous."

Defense mechanisms are essential for a balanced emotional life, so we don't want to strip them away willy-nilly. For example, it may be wise to stay in denial about a partner's affair until you're ready to deal with it. Becoming overwhelmed and unable to function in daily life serves no useful end. Also, some transitory emotional pain *does* go away if we block it out of our minds—and if it never returns, so much the better. We just don't want our psychological defenses to control us or complicate our lives.

Stepping on the hedonic treadmill of seeking pleasure and avoiding pain may *sometimes* be a good thing too. For example, if you don't pursue what you like, how can you ever be happy? Who else will satisfy your needs for you, in the short or long term, or even *know* what it takes to make you happy? For most adults, the days are long gone when other people can anticipate our needs better than we can. We need to take responsibility for our own happiness, and pleasure points the way. Hopefully, however, we'll choose longer term pleasures, such as the joy we feel from maintaining a healthy body, enriching the mind, and being helpful to others.

It's critical to know when the instinctive habits of seeking pleasure and avoiding pain are causing us more trouble than they're worth. Usually when we engage in these activities, stress is not far behind. We suffer when we don't get what we want, when we lose what we had, and when we get what we did *not* want. The ability to see things as they are, with acceptance, gets us through.

STAGES OF ACCEPTANCE

The process of turning toward discomfort occurs in stages; there's a progressive softening, or nonresistance, in the face of suffering.

After an initial bout of aversion, we start the process with curiosity about the problem and, if all goes well, end with a full embrace of whatever is occurring in our lives. The process is usually slow and natural. It makes no sense to advance to the next stage until you're entirely comfortable with where you are at the moment. The stages are:

1. *Aversion*—resistance, avoidance, rumination
2. *Curiosity*—turning toward discomfort with interest
3. *Tolerance*—safely enduring
4. *Allowing*—letting feelings come and go
5. *Friendship*—embracing, seeing hidden value

Our first, instinctive reaction to uncomfortable feelings is always *aversion*. For example, we avert our gaze when we see something unpleasant. Aversion can also take the form of mental entanglement or rumination—trying to figure out how to remove the feeling. After a while, when aversion doesn't work, we enter stage 2: *curiosity*. "What *is* that feeling?" "When does it happen?" "What does it mean?" When we know what we're dealing with, and if the pain doesn't go away, we may enter stage 3: *tolerance*. Tolerance means "enduring" emotional pain, but we're still resisting it and wishing it would go away. As our resistance erodes, we enter the fourth stage—*allowing*—letting difficult feelings come and go on their own. Finally, as our lives adapt and deepen, we may find ourselves in the *friendship* stage, where we actually see hidden value in our predicament. The story of a dear friend of mine, Brenda, helps illustrate what it's like to move through these stages.

Brenda and her husband, Doug, had two children. Their son, Zach, 3 years younger than his sister, was born with a congenital heart defect. When Brenda's family traveled to far-off places like Australia and Hawaii, Zach sometimes had a heart attack. He was a joyful, energetic boy despite his heart condition and the medications he was taking, but at 9 years old he died in his sleep. That was 19 years ago.

Stage 1: Aversion

The loss of a young child is an unspeakable agony. Although Brenda and Doug knew that Zach might not live long, nothing could prepare them for this. It was an "emotional tsunami." At the funeral, Brenda's nervous system was so overwrought that she lost her peripheral vision. She took to her bed after sitting shiva for 7 days, the Jewish custom of mourning. On rare occasions when she went out to the grocery store, Brenda felt like a foreigner, observing in a detached manner how people quibbled on the checkout line when they couldn't find their favorite type of pasta. Brenda was hiding deep within herself.

Stage 2: Curiosity

At some point, the thought occurred to Brenda, "If I just gave up, I could die." That seemed like a relief, but then she was seized with terror: "What about my daughter? What would she do? I can either succumb to my misery or make a choice." Brenda was gradually waking up to her predicament. "Feeling bad can be dangerous," she observed.

Stage 3: Tolerance

After 2 weeks, Brenda chose to get out of bed. "I made a choice to live for my daughter." As a child, Brenda had been her own mother's caregiver, so she certainly didn't want to burden her daughter by being incapacitated with grief. "I have to be a mother. Life is for the living," Brenda told herself. She explained to me later on, "The only salve for the misery was to help other people."

Stage 4: Allowing

Brenda describes herself as an "intellectual sort of person" who solves problems by thinking them through—"If your approach isn't working, try a new one"—but she was completely unprepared for this level of sadness. She and Doug kept their grief contained at a safe level by going to Zach's grave no more than twice a year and by occasionally taking out Zach's belongings and looking at them. "Did you know that the smell of his bathrobe goes away after 5 months?" The couple began allowing in more of the pain as they cried together during these "visits."

Psychologically, Brenda kept a loving relationship alive with Zach. She didn't want to let that go, nor did she need to. Brenda found that whenever she felt grief, she felt close to Zach. She also felt close when she had a wave of gratitude for having known Zach. Brenda was in psychotherapy at the time, so she asked her therapist, "Is it okay to have a living relationship with a dead person?" Her therapist replied, "Why not? Grief and gratitude are forms of love." Brenda was trusting her intuition to stay in a healthy relationship with Zach.

Stage 5: Friendship

When I met Brenda 17 years after Zach died, she said to me, "The pain of Zach's death has connected me to all mothers since the beginning of time who have lost children." Two years later, she was on a meditation retreat in which the teacher invited the students to "get in touch with their suffering." Brenda heard an inner voice that said, "I don't do that!" Then the teacher said, "If you can't be fully present with the difficult moments, chances are you won't be present with the best moments of your life either." At that moment, Brenda realized she'd been holding on to grief and "Maybe I don't need that anymore?" Without having spoken a word of this to her now 32-year-old daughter, 1 week later she received a call from her daughter asking for a referral to a counselor to speak about her brother's death. Not only was Brenda learning to befriend her own pain, but perhaps it invisibly prompted her daughter to do the same. Brenda told me, "It has taken me all this time to realize I can love fully without hurting."

This story illustrates what it's like to gradually soften our resistance to unbearable emotional pain. The stages don't necessarily occur in linear order; some days we drop back, and some days we leap forward. The deeper the sorrow, the longer it takes to pass through the stages of acceptance. Trying to rush the process is not helpful though, as it's a sure sign that we're trying to push away pain rather than cultivate acceptance. This book is designed to show you how to cultivate acceptance, especially *self*-acceptance, one day at a time.

FROM ACCEPTANCE TO SELF-COMPASSION

The mental health field is discovering the importance of accepting emotional pain. Ordinarily, when a person comes to therapy saying "I'm stressed out," the therapist tries to help him or her reduce the stress, perhaps by teaching relaxation skills. Therapists are very obliging that way. Sometimes they try to change distorted thinking that seems to make a person depressed (for example, "I'm stupid," or "I'll always be abandoned in the end"). These strategies fit into the category of "Tell me the problem and we'll fix it." In essence, therapists and clients unwittingly join forces, trying to uproot negative experience.

These approaches have met with reasonable success. Recent research indicates, however, that the healing mechanisms behind successful therapy are not what we thought they were: it's the process of establishing a new *relationship* with our thoughts and feelings, rather than directly challenging them, that makes the difference. This new relationship is less avoidant, less entangled, more accepting, more compassionate, and more aware. Leaning into our problems with open eyes and an open heart—with awareness and compassion—is the process by which we get emotional relief.

What's Acceptance?

As discussed earlier, "acceptance" covers a range of experiences, including curiosity, tolerance, willingness, and friendship. The opposite of acceptance is resistance. Whereas resistance creates suffering, acceptance alleviates it.

Acceptance doesn't mean tolerating bad behavior. It's opening emotionally to what's happening within us *in the present moment.* If you're in a painful relationship, acceptance doesn't mean you're saying "yes" to the entire relationship. Rather, it means acknowledging "This hurts!" I've seen many people make changes in their lives—relationships, eating habits, jobs—when they're in contact with how bad a situation or behavior makes them feel. Acceptance is not resignation or stagnation; change naturally follows acceptance.

But we need to know *what* we're accepting. Without awareness, we can become overly accommodating in our acceptance, like voting for a political candidate about whom we know very little. Blind acceptance can also devolve into sentimentality—sugarcoating reality. These are not examples of acceptance at all and will eventually lead to more suffering. I use "acceptance" in this book to refer to a conscious choice to experience our sensations, feelings, and thoughts *just as they are,* moment to moment.

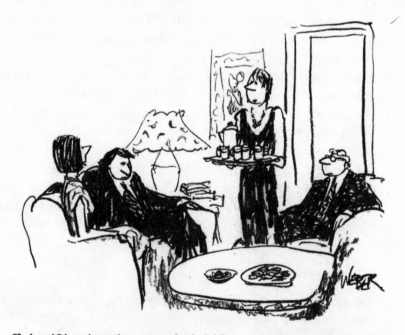

"Jack and I have learned to accept each other's idiosyncrasies, like my passion for cashew brittle, and his going out every night and not coming home until dawn."

What's Self-Compassion?

Self-compassion is a form of acceptance. Whereas acceptance usually refers to what's happening *to* us—accepting a feeling or a thought—self-compassion is acceptance of the *person* to whom it's happening. It's acceptance of ourselves while we're in pain.

Both acceptance and self-compassion seem to happen more easily after we've given up the struggle to feel better. This is known in Alcoholics Anonymous as the "gift of desperation." When everything you've tried has failed, you'll probably be more receptive to acceptance and self-compassion. Although you may still *want* to feel better, you doubt that anything will help you anymore. Your faith is nearly gone; the mind has exhausted its possibilities.

This is an opportunity to move from mental work to heart work. Self-compassion has a distinctly nonintellectual and noneffortful feel to it. If we can find ourselves in the midst of suffering and acknowledge the depth of our struggle, the heart begins to soften automatically. We stop trying to feel better and instead discover sympathy for ourselves. We start caring for ourselves *because* we're suffering.

There's an important distinction between "care" and "cure." Cure is what we try to do when we have some way to fix a problem. Care is what we can still do when all efforts at curing have failed. It's like attending to a dying person; we let go of the struggle and tenderly join in the experience of dying. In *emotional* life, the sooner we stop struggling to fix things, the better. Paradoxically, then, care leads to cure.

Compassion comes from the Latin roots *com* (with) and *pati* (suffer), or to "suffer with." When we offer genuine compassion, we join a person in his or her suffering. Being compassionate means that we recognize when someone is in pain, we abandon our fear of or resistance to it, and a natural feeling of love and kindness flows toward the suffering individual. The experience of compassion is complete abandonment of the inclination to resist emotional discomfort. It's *full* acceptance: of the person, of the pain, and of our own reactions to the pain.

Self-compassion is simply giving the same kindness to ourselves that we would give to others. As noted in the Introduction, it's a small shift in the direction of our attention that can make all the difference in our lives, both when we're in intense pain and as we negotiate the travails of daily life. We all have an instinct for self-compassion, perhaps forgotten or suppressed, that's even stronger than the instinct to resist suffering. Fortunately, self-compassion can be cultivated by anyone.

LET IT BE EASY

If these ideas seem remote or confusing, please don't be put off. When you practice them, they'll make more sense. The following chapters will lead you step by step until you can experience self-compassion whenever you need it.

Chapters 2 and 3 will introduce *mindfulness,* or how to recognize what's going on inside you, moment to moment, with kindly aware-ness. Most of us are too caught up in the details of our lives even to be aware when we're suffering. We need to locate the problem—the thorn in the heart—before we can implement a solution. Chapter 2 will show you how to become more aware of your body, safely and compassionately, and Chapter 3 will expand that awareness to the world of emotions. Then, starting in Chapter 4, you'll learn how to cultivate *self-compassion.*

Don't expect to do a lot of work. A patient of mine once said about self-compassion, "It's not about *fighting,* so it's not as difficult as I thought it would be." You might, however, occasionally catch yourself practicing an exercise with grim determination. That's to be expected—old habits die hard. Try to recognize when you're straining and see if you can do the same thing more enjoyably. We're not trying to add anything to our lives; we're subtracting. It's about giving up the tension we unconsciously impose on ourselves to con-trol or manipulate our experience.

The *principles* of mindfulness and self-compassion are at least as important as the techniques you're about to learn. The rationale behind the techniques has to be clear. For example, if you feel an exercise isn't working, maybe you're practicing "self-improvement" rather than "self-acceptance." You need to know the difference. Once you've thoroughly understood the meaning of mindfulness and self-compassion, you can modify the exercises given in this book to fit any situation you encounter.

Finally, if you ever find yourself doubting that you can become more self-compassionate, stop and bring a little kindness to yourself in that very moment. You'll be practicing the essence of what this book has to offer.

TRY THIS: Waiting on Yourself

We usually attend to *others*—what they're feeling, saying, and doing. It's rare that we wait on ourselves with equal care and consideration. Let's try that now. This exercise takes only 5 minutes. You can't do it wrong.

Choose a quiet place, sit comfortably, close your eyes, and notice what it feels like to be in your body. Just be with the physical sensations in your body as they come and go, without choosing to pay attention to any particular one. If it's a pleasant one, feel it and let it go. If it's an unpleasant one, also feel it and let it go. Perhaps you feel warmth in your hands, pressure on the seat, tingling in the forehead? Notice those sensations as a mother would gaze at a newborn baby, wondering what it's feeling. Just notice whatever arises, one sensation after another. Take your time.

After 5 minutes, gently open your eyes.

2

listening to your body

It is just simple attention that allows us to truly listen
to the sound of the bird, to see deeply the glory of
an autumn leaf, to touch the heart of another and be
touched.
—CHRISTINA FELDMAN AND JACK KORNFIELD,
meditation teachers

t's not easy living in a human body, but fortunately we have what
it takes. We're endowed with the human faculties of awareness
and compassion. The first step toward being at ease within the
body is to pay attention to it. We need to know what ails us. Then
we can respond with compassion.

When we're suffering, it's not always immediately apparent what
the problem is. If I get fired from my job, for example, I might think
that I was treated unfairly and that my boss held a personal grudge
against me. Sleepless in the middle of the night, I'll despair that I'm
a poor provider for my family and imagine taking revenge on my
boss. Where am I, the sensitive, wounded soul, in all this? Gone!
I've run off into my mind—taken the elevator to the top floor—and
blocked out my feelings of fear and sadness. I'm arguing with the
world about my personal value and scheming about the future. It's

36

often like that when we suffer. We can't find ourselves in the crowd of thoughts and feelings that swirls around in our heads.

Mindfulness is a special type of awareness that can keep us anchored safely in our bodies when the going gets tough. It can grow into a way of life that protects us from unnecessary suffering. When we're mindful, there's less need to escape unpleasant experience—there's a little breathing room around it. This chapter will explain what mindfulness is and what it isn't in a way that will clarify how resisting the urge to escape pain sets us free. I'll offer a few easy mindfulness techniques.

THE MINDFUL PATH

Mindfulness has to be experienced to be known. It can't be expressed adequately in words. A moment of mindfulness is a kind of awareness that comes *before* words, such as the twinkling of stars before we call them the Big Dipper or a dash of red at the door before we recognize it as a friend wearing a new red dress. Our brains go through this preverbal level of awareness all the time, but we're normally too caught up in the drama of everyday life to notice.

Poetry captures the simple experience of mindfulness:

Every day
   I see or I hear
      something
         that more or less

kills me
   with delight,
      that leaves me
         like a needle

in the haystack
   of light.
      It was what I was born for—
         to look, to listen,

to lose myself
    inside this soft world—
        to instruct myself
            over and over

in joy,
    and acclamation.
        Nor am I talking
            about the exceptional,

the fearful, the dreadful,
    the very extravagant—
        but of the ordinary,
            the common, the very drab,

the daily presentations.
    Oh, good scholar,
        I say to myself,
            how can you help

but grow wise
    with such teachings
        as these—
            the untrimmable light

of the world,
    the ocean's shine,
        the prayers that are made
            out of grass?

Mary Oliver reminds us in this poem, "Mindful," how simple perceptions like the dance of light on a blade of wet grass can fill us with delight.

The definition of mindfulness that I find particularly useful is from meditation teacher Guy Armstrong: "Knowing what you are experiencing *while* you're experiencing it." Mindfulness is moment-to-moment awareness. There's freedom in mindfulness because paying attention to our stream of perceptions, rather than our *interpreta-tions* of them, makes every moment fresh and alive. Life becomes a festival to the senses when we're mindful. Consider this moment of ordinary life in a poem by Linda Bamber:

Suddenly the city
I live in seems interesting
as if I were on vacation here
and feeling indulgent
towards the human race, its way of
living in cities and
tearing up roads so the traffic has to be
re-routed around a collapsing white mesh barrier
as in this intersection here.
The people of this city
walking back and forth on the sidewalks
each one having gotten up and dressed this morning
look like this, this
movie, almost, of people crossing the street.
The questions,
is this scene in any way rewarding to look at?
e.g., architecturally, in terms of city spaces and human interest; and
are things diverse enough here? and
are these people, in general,
older or younger than I am? just now are
in abeyance. In their absence is this
pleasant sense that there are many cities in the world
and this is one of them.
It rained earlier. I think I'll go see the monks
make a sand mandala on the Esplanade; and
who knows, later I might get a sandwich.

Mindfulness has a quality of *being in the now*, a sense of freedom, of perspective, of being connected, not judging, of flowing through the day. When we're mindful, we're less likely to want life to be other than it is, at least for the moment.

Some people seem to be more mindful than others, but no mat-ter where our starting point is, we can increase mindfulness through practice. And you don't need to be a monk or a poet to benefit from mindfulness training. You don't even need to be calm to be mindful; you just need to make a personal commitment to be aware. You can wake up to your day-to-day life at any time or place by recognizing what's going on in and around yourself. Ask yourself: Am I feeling confused, bored, elated, stressed, or peaceful? Can I sense tension in my stomach, warmth on my cheeks? Am I worrying about the future, what will happen when I visit my father later? Is that the sound of fluttering leaves on a poplar tree? Any awareness in present time can be a moment of mindfulness and a relief from our usual tension-producing mental machinations.

The opposite of mindfulness is mind*less*ness, which happens, for example, when you:

- Forget someone's name right after you are introduced

- Don't remember what you just walked into the kitchen for

- Eat when you're not hungry

- Fret about being late when you're stuck in a traffic jam

- Act like a child when you visit your parents

- Drive for an hour on the highway with hardly any memory of it

These are times when we're preoccupied, unaware of what we're thinking, feeling, or doing, and reacting as if we're on autopilot. You may have noticed how mindlessly we spend most of our lives!

Mindlessness is not a problem if the movie we're playing in our heads is sweet and enjoyable, but sometimes it's scary and we'd like nothing better than to get up and leave the theater. Our attention gets kidnapped by our suffering. This was the situation for one of my patients, George.

By all outward appearances, George was doing well in life. He had a job he liked, he had recently bought a home, he had a partner who loved him, and he could delight his friends with his skill on the guitar. But the more he flourished, the more George found that memories from his difficult childhood plagued him. He had grown up in a poor and abusive household, and his beloved sister had committed suicide when she was 16 years old. George couldn't keep himself from sobbing whenever something good happened to him, such as getting a raise at work, buying a new car, or going on vacation. He thought about his sad childhood with his sister and how she had never had a chance to enjoy her life. His regret would not allow him to be happy. Sometimes George had flashback memories when he read news reports of battered children. His wife became concerned that she was losing her connection to George, who seemed to become increasingly preoccupied with his past as good things came their way.

George really wanted to remain close to his wife, who couldn't help losing her patience with him at times. One day, while walking on the beach, preoccupied as usual, George noticed a beautiful round stone. He picked it up, rolled it around in his hand, rubbed it on his face, and enjoyed its cool, smooth texture on his cheeks. Since George was a collector, he absent-mindedly slipped the stone into his coat pocket. When George got home, he rediscovered the rock when he emptied his pockets. Again, it felt good to the touch: smooth, cool, and round. George noticed how rubbing it with his fingers soothed him. He dubbed it his "here-and-now stone" and kept it with him always. Whenever George found that he had a flashback memory of his childhood and didn't want to get lost in it, he took the stone out of his pocket and ran his fingers over it.

Without any outside instruction, George had stumbled upon a way of managing his mind through mindfulness—bringing his mind into sensory awareness of the here-and-now. At first, George used his here-and-now stone to shift his attention *away* from what was bothering him and into the present moment. Later on, when the present moment and his stone became a reliable place of refuge when he was emotionally overwhelmed, George felt the courage to turn *toward* his traumatic memories, exploring them in detail. Mindfulness is both knowing where our mind is from moment to moment *and* directing our attention in skillful ways.

An attitude of openheartedness is necessary for mindfulness to be healing. Like a mother gazing at an infant child, we can look at something for a long period of time if it's something we love or if we feel loved and supported while looking. It's not possible to be aware of anything for very long if we're disgusted by it. We can experience the exquisite beauty of a rose, or a piece of music, or ourselves only if we're emotionally open. That's the spirit in which we practice mindfulness.

BEGINNING TO PRACTICE MINDFULNESS

If you did the "Waiting on Yourself" exercise at the end of the last chapter, you've already had a taste of mindfulness. Your mind was in a relatively receptive state, aware of a series of perceptions without needing to compare, judge, label, or evaluate them. It's easy to live in our own minds if we simply notice what comes and goes. Problems occur when we unconsciously recoil at discomfort, grasp for pleasure, and slip into mental fantasies about how things should be. Every one of us, without exception, soon discovers that a simple exercise like sitting still for a few minutes and allowing our thoughts to come and go is anything but easy.

TRY THIS: *Mindfulness of Sound*

This exercise takes only 5 minutes. Find a reasonably quiet place, one in which you won't be distracted by the TV, music, or people talking.

- Sit in a relaxed, comfortable position with a straight spine. Let your eyes close, fully or partially.

- Imagine that your ears are like satellite dishes picking up any sounds in the environment. Just sit and receive sound vibrations. You don't need to label the sounds, you don't need to *like* the sounds, and you don't need to keep your attention with any particular sound— just hear whatever presents itself to you. Let the sounds come and go, one after another. Don't try to search out sounds around you. Let them come to you.

- When you notice that your mind has wandered away on a train of thought, as it inevitably will, simply return to the task of listening.
- After 5 minutes, slowly open your eyes.

You might have noticed how relaxing it can be to simply pay attention to sounds, perhaps even more comforting than other methods you may be familiar with, such as relaxation training or self-hypnosis. That's because you let go of whatever was on your mind, including the task of "relaxing," which may paradoxically keep you on edge. You were just "being" with the symphony of sound around you.

Maybe you also discovered that you added a few extra tasks to the simple act of listening. For example, you might have labeled the sounds: "car," "child laughing," "door shutting." That's more work. You might also have wished you were in a more beautiful place, like the countryside, with sweeter sounds. That creates a little stress. And your mind probably started wandering in a very short time; perhaps you wondered if you were doing the exercise correctly, or you thought about buying a quieter air conditioner. Each of these automatic mental functions—labeling, judging, wandering mind—makes listening a little harder than it needs to be.

If you can, try the same exercise again. You could make a mental note of judging, labeling, and thinking when these mental functions kick in and then return to the sounds. Say to yourself "labeling," when you notice you're labeling, or "judging" when you're judging, and "thinking" when you catch yourself lost in thought.

Anchoring Your Mind

The mind needs an anchor. Most of our mental suffering arises when our minds jump around from one subject to another, which is exhausting, or when we're preoccupied with unhappy thoughts and feelings. When we notice that the mind is behaving in this way, we need to give it an anchor—a place to go that's neutral and unwavering. That's what George did when he rubbed his here-and-now stone and what you did when you returned your attention, again and again, to the sounds in your environment. Anchoring calms the mind.

The most common anchor for the mind is the breath. There are good reasons for this:

- The breath is happening 24 hours a day.
- It's easy to notice because it creates a slight movement in the body.
- It's familiar, so it can be a safe refuge from the storms of daily life.
- It operates automatically, without any personal effort.
- It's our most loyal friend, accompanying us from birth to death.

Awareness of the breath is an excellent way to gather your attention and bring yourself into the present moment.

Some people find it difficult to focus on the breath. People who've endured physical trauma may not like being reminded of their bodies because it brings up bad memories. Those with health anxiety find that focusing on any part of the body triggers new worries. Detail-oriented or compulsive types of people may discover that when they focus on the breath their attention grips it too tightly and they experience shortness of breath. People who don't like the way their bodies look or feel may find that attention to the breath brings them too close to their bodies in general.

If you have any of these experiences, give yourself a different anchor. The only prerequisite is that it be readily available. Some people like to use a word as an anchor—perhaps one that has special meaning (see "Centering Meditation" in Appendix B). Other choices could be the feeling of the floor under your feet, your hands folded in your lap, or an area of your body such as the heart region or a point between your eyes. If it's difficult to bring your attention *inside* your body, choose an object on the surface of your body or outside it. Whatever you choose as an anchor, over time it will become like a very close friend.

The following exercise shows how to use the breath as an anchor, but feel free to substitute a different object for your attention.

TRY THIS: *Mindfulness of Breathing*

This exercise takes 15 minutes. Please find a quiet, comfortable place to sit. Sit in a way that your bones are supporting the muscles and you don't need any effort to remain in one position for the whole exercise. To do this, try keeping your back straight and gently supported, with your shoulder blades slightly dropped and your chin gently tucked toward your chest.

- Take three, slow, easy deep breaths to relax and let go of whatever burdens you're carrying around. Then let your eyelids gently close, or partially close, whichever makes you feel more comfortable.

- Form an image of yourself sitting down. Note your posture on the chair as if you were seeing yourself from the outside. Let your body and mind be just as they are.

- Now bring your attention to your breathing. Pay attention to *where* you notice your breathing most strongly. Some people feel it at the nostrils, perhaps as a cool breeze on the upper lip. Other people can feel the chest rising and falling. Still others feel the breath most clearly in the abdomen, as the belly expands with every in-breath and contracts with every out-breath. Gently explore your body and discover where your breathing is easiest to notice.

- Now discover *when* you feel your breath more strongly—when you exhale or when you inhale. If they're about equal, choose one. (To simplify the instructions, I'll assume for the rest of this exercise and throughout the book that you chose exhaling and that the location you selected was the nostrils.)

- Pay attention to the feeling of each exhalation. Feel the air coming out of your nostrils each time you exhale. Then take a little vacation as your body inhales. Let your entire experience just *be* as you wait. Then feel your breath as your body exhales again.

- Let your body breathe *you*—it does that automatically anyway. Simply pay attention to the sensation of the air in your nose each time you exhale, one breath after another.

- Your mind will wander away from the sensation of the breath many times every minute. Don't worry about how often your mind wanders. Gently return to the feeling of your out-breath at the nostrils when you notice that your mind has wandered.

- You might be using a watch to keep track of time. Sneak a peek at your watch, and when you have a few minutes left, loosen your focus on the nostrils and allow yourself to feel your whole upper body move with each breath. Don't bother thinking too much about it. Just feel your body, alive and moving, as you breathe.

- After 15 minutes, gently open your eyes, looking downward. Savor the stillness of the moment before moving on.

You've probably noticed how busy the mind is. It's very difficult to find the breath amid the clamor of competing thoughts and feelings. No sooner do we focus fully on one out-breath than the mind is off and running on a new train of thought. Perhaps you thought, "Oh, that's a nice breath," and as you inhaled you were already thinking of another sensation in the body or what you were going to do later in the day. When the object of our attention is repetitive and neutral, rather than novel and compelling, our brains quickly start sorting through other business.

Mindfulness of the breath cultivates focus on a single object, but you shouldn't expect your attention to remain unwaveringly with the breath. That's not how the brain operates. Just return your attention again and again to the breath when you notice your mind has wandered. Nothing more. It's like the Zen saying "If you fall down six times, get up seven." When people say, "I can't medi-

The "Default Network"

In 2001, Debra Gusnard and Marcus Raichle identified a whole dis-crete network of brain regions—the default network—that is active when the mind is at rest and that becomes *in*active when the mind is engaged in a task. When the mind wanders in meditation, it's in default mode. The default network operates in the background, linking our past to the future and providing us with a sense of "self." We're usually aware of the default network only when it has failed, such as in patients with Alzheimer's disease who appear "mentally empty."

Giuseppe Pagnoni and colleagues at Emory University observed the default network during meditation using fMRI (functional mag-netic resonance imaging). They asked two groups—Zen practitioners with more than 3 years of daily practice and a comparison group that never meditated—to focus on their breath, to occasionally decide whether a string of letters presented to them was a real English word ("conceptual processing"), and then to return to their breathing. Conceptual processing activated the default network. Zen practi-tioners were able to return to the breath and turn off the default network more quickly than the comparison group; they could rapidly abandon the stream of associations that spontaneously arose after thinking about the meaning of words. The authors speculate that this ability may help alleviate psychological conditions characterized by rumination, such as obsessive–compulsive disorder, anxiety disor-ders, and major depression.

It's not clear why we have a default network. Gusnard and Raichle speculate that it's crucial for human functioning. For example, the dorsal medial prefrontal cortex, a brain region that is active when we monitor our own thoughts, speech, and actions or those of others, is in the default network. It appears that this part of the default net-work is not just involved in "free association" and "mind wandering," but also when we're preparing for the future. Meditators should not blame themselves when their minds wander—when their brains do what they evolved to do while at rest.

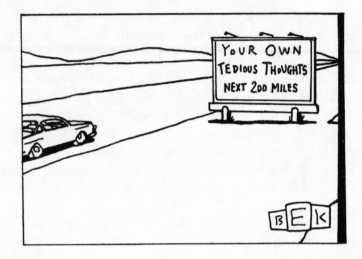

tate," they're usually referring to the erroneous assumption that they should be concentrating better. Distractions are a part of meditation. Each moment of recognizing distraction actually should be welcomed rather than used as an occasion for self-criticism, because it shows that you've just "woken up" from daydreaming.

Daydreaming can sometimes be a good thing, perhaps a source of creative inspiration, much like Sigmund Freud was referring to when he described our night dreams as the "royal road to the unconscious." The key is to *know* when we're daydreaming and to wake up occasionally. Unfortunately, most of the time our attention is lost in our daydreams and we suffer from stressful preoccupations—"Do I look fat?" "That was dumb!" When we return to the breath, we have a moment of respite. There are no issues when we're in the present moment. When you're upset, see what happens when you take a walk and focus only on the sensations of your feet on the sidewalk. No past, no future ... no problem.

If you find that your stress level *increases* when you do the mindfulness of breathing exercise, try to do it in a new way. First of all, let go of the need to get it right. (You'll *never* get it right—and you'll never get it wrong.) Learn to work harmoniously with the mind as it is. The mind will always dredge up another memory or feeling that will disturb your concentration, so don't despair when that happens. We don't meditate to improve ourselves; we meditate to *end* our compulsive striving to do everything better. The sign of a seasoned practitioner is the willingness to return to the breath, again and again, without judgment, for *decades*.

Anchoring your attention in the breath does more than cultivate a focused, calm mind—it allows you to *see how the mind works*. It's like holding a camera steady to take a picture. From the three exercises presented in this book so far, you've already learned how easily the mind wanders, compares, judges, and labels whatever it perceives. The longer you spend in meditation, the more you'll discover about your mind. You'll also discover a lot about *yourself*: your emotions, your memories, and how you react to different circumstances.

Knowing that you can always take refuge in your anchor will give you courage to explore your mind. It's like the child who hides behind his mother's skirt when he's feeling timid; knowing that we can calm ourselves by returning to the anchor/breath enables us to peek back into our turbulent inner worlds.

MINDFULNESS OF THE BODY

The body is the foundation of mindfulness training. We live in a body, so to appreciate the fullness of life we need to experience the body fully. We shouldn't think that the body is less important than the mind when we practice mindfulness. Anything occurring in the present is a suitable object of mindful awareness. Since the body is relatively slow and stable, it's an excellent vantage point for observing our mind and emotions. The problem with trying to be aware of thoughts in mindfulness meditation is that thoughts occur so quickly that we can hardly keep track of them; they're ancient history the moment we notice them. The mind also becomes quickly absorbed in its own ramblings when it observes itself. It's much easier to remain aware of the present moment when we focus on the body.

We've already begun practicing mindfulness of the body by focusing on the breath. Now let's open the field of awareness to body sensations *around* the breath.

TRY THIS: *Mindfulness of Body Sensations*

This exercise takes about 20 minutes. Please begin by finding a comfortable, stable position, close your eyes, and take three relaxing breaths.

- Form an image of yourself. Note your posture on the chair as if you were seeing yourself from the outside.

- Find your breath within your body and practice mindfulness of breathing for a few minutes. Let your body breathe itself while you feel every out-breath, one after another.

- After a few minutes, release your attention from your breath and open your awareness to your entire body—to the space within the skin. Your body is vibrating with activity at every moment. Let your attention be called to whatever sensation predominates. Simply notice one, two, or three sensations in succession, such as your beating heart, moist feet, tight neck, warm hands, cool forehead, clenched jaw, or the touch of your body on the chair.

- Let each sensation be just as it is. If you feel discomfort, incline toward it gently and softly in your mind.

- Let your attention be with body sensations as long as it's naturally drawn there and then return to your breath. You can return to your breath anytime you need to gather and stabilize your attention.

- Then open your awareness again to whatever body sensations call to you—whatever you feel most strongly. Take it slow and easy. The task is to remain with sensations occurring in the present moment, not to identify as many sensations as possible.

- For the remaining 10 to 15 minutes, let yourself feel your breathing and then feel any other predominant sensations in the body. Go back and forth between the breath and other sensations in a relaxed, leisurely manner. Notice your breathing alongside the other sensations going on in your body. Be fully embodied, breathing and feeling.

• Gently open your eyes.

Did you feel yourself relax when you returned to the breath after being aware of the other sensations in the body? Perhaps you had the opposite experience—that focusing only on your breathing felt constricting and full-body awareness was a relief?

Mindfulness meditation is commonly a dance between single-focus and open-field awareness. When our attention is too tight around the breath, causing stress, we can relax by opening our awareness to other perceptions. Alternatively, when our attention is swept up in the tornado of events continually occurring in the body or mind, we can find shelter from the storm in one-pointed attention to the breath.

SHOULD I MEDITATE?

There are two categories of mindfulness meditation: formal and informal. "Formal" mindfulness meditation is when we dedicate time—usually half an hour or longer—to being mindful of what we're sensing, feeling, and thinking. "Informal" meditation is when we take a brief, mindful moment in the midst of our busy lives. Both approaches can be practiced while sitting down, standing, walking, eating—anywhere and anytime. The difference between formal and informal meditation is mainly a matter of time and purpose.

Each person should decide for him- or herself whether it makes sense to establish a formal meditation practice. Formal practice is more intensive, which generally transforms the mind at a deeper level: it yields deeper insights into the nature of mind and our personal conditioning. If you wish to do formal meditation, it should be enjoyable and it should fit your temperament and lifestyle. Most people don't want to squeeze yet another activity into their busy schedules. Nor should they. This book is not written for people who want to become meditators, although some readers might develop a taste for it. The formal meditation practices here are offered primarily so you can have a direct experience of mindfulness and self-compassion, and they can be used as a model for practicing more informally.

Formal meditation is never an end in itself; life itself is the real practice. It's hard to stay conscious and aware amid the flood of sensory impressions and emotional reactions we encounter in daily life. Consider your mind state on a morning when your baby daughter has been sick all night, you have to make a presentation at the office in 3 hours, the freezer door was left open all night and ice cream is dripping on the floor, and your babysitter is on vacation. Many parents would find themselves crying on the kitchen floor. Maintaining presence of mind to handle problems calmly and efficiently is a skill that grows with meditation practice. If you spend a chunk of time every day exploring your inner experience in formal meditation, the same kind of compassionate self-monitoring is more likely to continue throughout the day, even during the worst of times.

Formal mindfulness meditation especially helps us figure out how to *live with discomfort*—to inhabit our bodies in a way that doesn't turn everyday physical and emotional pain into a larger problem. Depending on how you're feeling from moment to moment, you might focus your attention on the breath, explore a body ache, return to the breath, sense an emotion, find the emotion in the body, breathe, soften the body a little, breathe, listen to sounds in the environment, return to the breath, and so on. This practice gives us, in Jon Kabat-Zinn's words, the freedom to "respond" rather than "react." We can make wise choices about our lives: "Shall I eat that snack? Should I argue with my spouse right now? Is this a good time to act on a sexual urge?"

How much formal meditation is generally recommended? The usual length of time is 30 to 45 minutes daily. That amount has been shown to increase well-being and even enhance the immune

Training Your Brain

In 2003, Richard Davidson, Jon Kabat-Zinn, and colleagues found that 8 weeks of mindfulness meditation training (mindfulness-based stress reduction [MBSR]), 1 hour daily, 6 days a week, produced lasting changes in the brain and the immune system. Twenty-five stressed-out biotech employees were trained to meditate, and they were compared to 16 people who received no training at all. After the meditation training, everyone was asked to write down one of the most positive experiences of their lives and one of the most negative experiences. EEG recordings were made of their brains before and after the writing exercise. Their blood was also drawn to measure how many antibodies they produced in response to a flu vaccine.

EEG recordings showed that meditators had increased activation in the left side of the frontal region of their brains, an area associated with positive emotions. This brain activity was evident even when meditators wrote about *negative* experiences in their lives, suggesting that they had learned to adapt well to unpleasant mind states. Blood tests were given at 4 and 8 weeks after the flu vaccine was administered and meditators generated more antibodies than nonmeditators, demonstrating stronger immune systems. Interestingly, the number of flu antibodies correlated with left-sided brain activation among the meditators—more left frontal activation, more antibodies.

In 2008, David Creswell and colleagues also measured the impact of the MBSR program on immune functioning. They trained an ethnically diverse sample of 48 HIV-positive patients in the MBSR program and thereafter counted the number of CD4 T cells—the cells that are destroyed by the HIV virus. (CD4 T cells are considered the "brains" of the immune system that protect the body against attack.) Creswell and colleagues found that "the more mindfulness meditation classes people attended, the higher the CD4 T cells at the study's conclusion."

Charles Raison and colleagues at Emory University examined the effect of meditation on the inflammatory protein, interleukin-6. Chronic stress increases plasma concentrations of IL-6, and elevated IL-6 predicts illnesses such as vascular disease, diabetes, dementia, and depression. The researchers compared a group of students who completed 8 weeks of compassion meditation (with some mindfulness meditation) to a group that had twice-weekly health discussions. Afterwards, all students were put under stress in a public speaking and mental arithmetic challenge. No clear differences in IL-6 were found between the meditation and control groups. However, meditators who practiced more than average had significantly lower levels of IL-6 compared to their less zealous colleagues, suggesting that mind training can reduce inflammatory responses to stress.

system. Busy people are more likely to meditate for 20 minutes, once or twice a day, which is also good. Improvement appears to be "dose-dependent"—it depends on *how much* training is given.

Some parts of the brain even grow thicker when we meditate daily over a period of years. Sara Lazar and colleagues at Harvard University measured whether long-term mindfulness meditation can change the physical structure of the brain. They found that the prefrontal cortex and the right anterior insula—regions associated with attention, internal awareness, and sensory processing—were thicker in long-term meditators than in matched controls. Furthermore, cortical thickening correlated with years of meditation experience and seemed to offset thinning of the cerebral cortex that naturally occurs as we age.

The psychological mechanisms by which long-term mindfulness meditation translates into less suffering are under preliminary investigation. One hypothesis is that our difficult memories lose their edge if they arise when we're in a calm state of mind—"interoceptive exposure." Another is that we learn to regulate our attention, and knowing when and where to place our attention helps us regulate emotion. George did this by focusing on his here-and-now stone when he was overwhelmed by trauma flashbacks. Yet another potential mechanism of action for mindfulness meditation is "metacognition," the ability to step back and witness our thoughts and feelings rather than getting hijacked by them.

Perhaps the most compelling explanation for why mindfulness works is that, over time, we acquire beneficial insights about life. We discover how everything changes, how we create our own suffering when we *fight* change, and how we unconsciously cobble together a sense of "self." The latter insight is beneficial because most of our waking moments are spent vainly boosting or fearfully protecting our fragile egos from assault. (More is said about this baffling, yet important, topic near the end of Chapters 4 and 5.) When these insights about life become deep and abiding, they help us receive success and failure with equanimity, tolerate emotional pain knowing "this too will pass," and have the courage to seize each precious moment of our lives. In other words, intuitive insights derived from

What Mindfulness Is Not

- *Mindfulness is not trying to relax.* When we become aware of what's happening in our lives, it can be anything but relaxing, especially if we're stuck in a difficult situation. As we learn more about ourselves, however, we become less surprised by the feelings that arise within us. We develop a less reactive relationship to inner experience. We can recognize and let go of emotional storms more easily.

- *Mindfulness is not a religion.* Although mindfulness has been practiced by Buddhist nuns and monks for over 2,500 years, any purposeful activity that increases awareness of moment-to-moment experience is a mindfulness exercise. We can practice mindfulness as part of a religion or not. Modern scientific psychology considers mindfulness to be a core healing factor in psychotherapy.

- *Mindfulness is not about transcending ordinary life.* Mindfulness is making intimate contact with each moment of our lives, no matter how trivial or mundane. Simple things can become very special—extraordinarily ordinary—with this type of awareness. For example, the flavor of your food or the color of a rose will be enhanced if you pay close attention to it. Mindfulness is also about experiencing oneself more fully, not trying to bypass the mundane, ragged edges of our lives.

- *Mindfulness is not emptying the mind of thoughts.* The brain will always produce thoughts—that's what it does. Mindfulness allows us to develop a more harmonious relationship with our thoughts and feelings through a deep understanding of how the mind works. It may *feel* as if we have fewer thoughts, because we're not struggling with them so much.

- *Mindfulness is not difficult.* You shouldn't feel disheartened when you discover that your mind wanders incessantly. That's the nature of the mind. It's also the nature of the mind to eventually become aware of its wandering. Ironically, it's in the very moment when you despair that you're not mindful that you've become mindful. It's not possible to do this practice perfectly, nor is it possible to fail. That is why it's called a "practice."

- *Mindfulness is not escape from pain.* This is the toughest idea to accept because we rarely do anything without the wish to feel better. You *will* feel better with mindfulness and acceptance, but only by learning *not* to escape from pain. Pain is like an angry bull: When it's confined to a tight stall, it will be wild and try to escape. When it's in a wide-open field, it will calm down. Mindfulness makes emotional space for pain.

intensive meditation can help us establish a less defensive, more flex-ible, relationship to the world.

PRACTICING MINDFULNESS IN DAILY LIFE

Mindfulness in daily life is "informal" meditation practice. Short moments of mindful awareness can substantially reduce the stress that we accumulate throughout the day. And it feels good to just *be,* if only for a few seconds.

Informal practice means we choose to pay attention, on pur-pose, to what's occurring in the present moment. *Any moment-to-moment experience is a suitable object of mindfulness.* That could mean listening to birds, tasting your food, feeling the earth beneath your feet as you walk, noticing the grip of your hands on the steering wheel, scanning your body for physical sensations, or noticing your breathing. It could be as simple as wiggling your toes. The present moment liberates us from our preoccupations, never judges us, and is endlessly entertaining.

Don't underestimate the power of brief mindfulness exercises. A report in the psychological literature describes a 27-year-old man, James, who suffered from mild mental retardation and mental ill-ness. He was hospitalized several times for aggressive behavior. Dur-ing one hospitalization, James received mindfulness training twice a day for 5 days, plus assignments for another week. The training went like this:

- Stand or sit with your feet flat on the floor.
- Breathe normally.
- Think of something that leads to feeling angry.
- Shift your focus to your feet and wait until you feel calm.

James practiced this "soles of the feet" meditation whenever he became angry. One year later, his aggressive behavior had decreased significantly, he was able to stop taking all the medication he had been on, and his caregivers no longer considered him mentally ill.

Customizing Mindfulness Exercises

The most important thing to keep in mind when you tailor mindfulness exercises for yourself is to make them as pleasurable as possible. Mindful awareness comes naturally when we're enjoying ourselves.

All mindfulness exercises have three basic components:

- Stop
- Observe
- Return

Stop

First we need to stop what we're doing. If you're arguing on the phone, you can take a moment of silence. If you're caught in a traffic jam and worrying about being late, you might take a deep, conscious breath. *Slowing down* also facilitates mindfulness. If you eat more slowly, you'll be more aware of what you're eating, and you might even give your body a chance to tell you when you're full. When you reduce your walking speed, you'll see more of your surroundings.

Observe

Observing doesn't mean detachment or being overly objective. Instead, you want to be a "participant observer," intimately engaged with the experience. Life is bubbling within you and you're in the middle of it, yet you can observe.

If calming down is your wish, it helps to have a single point of observation, such as the breath. If you want to explore and understand what you're feeling at the moment, you can scan your body for sensations and perhaps label your emotions: "anger," "fear," "sadness." (Much more will be said about mindfulness of emotions in the following chapter.)

Return

When you notice that your attention has been swept away into daydreams, gently return it to the focal object. If you're in nature and wish to be more mindful of your surroundings, that may mean returning again and again to the sounds of the forest. If you're chopping vegetables, it's a safe bet that you'll want to pay attention to the distance between your finger and the blade of the knife. (The closer our fingers get to the blade, the easier mindfulness becomes!)

Conscious Breathing

Whenever you feel stuck or confused, you can begin making the situation workable by taking a mindful breath: just stop what you're doing and feel your breath. You can take a conscious breath anytime: in your car at a red light, during a business meeting, or while your child is having a tantrum. Let yourself be immersed in the nourishing experience of breathing. When you feel calmer and your mind has cleared, give yourself a chance to choose what to do next. Conscious breathing is the easiest, most common mindfulness technique; *remembering* to do it in the midst of our busy lives is the challenge.

Mindful Walking

Walking meditation is a delightful practice, especially if you've been sitting all day long and need a little exercise. You can practice walking as a formal, 20- to 30-minute meditation, or in spurts—as you walk to the bus stop or from your car to the grocery store. Anytime your feet hit the pavement, you can meditate. Of course, a meditative walk in the woods is a special way of opening to the beauty of nature.

TRY THIS: Mindful Walking

Plan to walk for 10 minutes or longer. Find a quiet place in your home where you can walk back and forth at least 20–30 feet at a time or in a circle. Make the decision to use the time to cultivate moment-to-moment kindly awareness.

- Stand still for a moment and anchor your attention in your body. Be aware of yourself in the standing posture. Feel your body.

- Start to walk slowly and deliberately. Notice how it feels to lift one foot, step forward, and place it down as the other foot begins to lift off the floor. Do the same with the other foot. Feel the sensations of lifting, stepping, and placing, over and over again. Feel free to use the words "lift," "step," "place" to focus your attention on the task.

- When your mind wanders, gently return to the physical sensations of walking. If you feel any urgency to move faster, simply note that and return to the sensations of walking.

- Do this with kindness and gratitude. Your relatively small feet are supporting your entire body; your hips are supporting your whole torso. Experience the marvel of walking.

- Move slowly and fluidly through space, being aware that you're walking. Some people find it easiest to keep their attention below the knees, or exclusively on the soles of the feet.

- When you reach the end of your walking space, pause a moment, take a conscious breath, remain anchored in your body, and reverse direction.

- At the end of the meditation period, invite yourself to be mindful of body sensations throughout the day. Notice the sensations of walking as you go on to your next activity.

Do this exercise first at home, walking very slowly, and later walk at a normal pace when outside in public. It can be very grounding to feel the earth beneath your feet, especially when you're in a hurry or emotionally upset. Some people prefer to just focus on their breathing while walking. That's fine too. As in all mindfulness exercises, feel free to experiment and discover what works best for you.

In the next chapter, we turn our attention to emotions: What are they? Where do they come from? How can you use mindfulness to deal with them, and why does it work?

3

bringing in difficult emotions

*How can emotions not be part of that singing life of grasses
and fish and oil tankers and subways and cats who wake us,
furious and smiling, in the middle of the brief summer night?*
—JANE HIRSHFIELD, *poet*

From the exercises in Chapter 2, you may have discovered the emotional relief that comes when you anchor your attention in the body. That's the first step toward regulating emotions: stabilizing attention. The next step is turning toward difficult emotions.

Why would we want to do that? Unfortunately, difficult feelings are a part of everyone's life, so we need to deal with them in the best possible way. We'll never be able to relax if we're fugitives from our own feelings. Some difficult emotions disappear on their own, like disappointment with your favorite baseball team or frustration over an unexpected car problem. Other feelings, like anger at a parent or fear following a car accident, may never quit. Relief only comes when we take a fresh look at those feelings and change our *relationship* to them.

Many emotions are "difficult," such as fear, anger, and hatred, but none are inherently "destructive." At the very least, difficult emotions provide information about what's happening inside and out. Emotions become destructive—leading to greater mental or physical suffering—when we cling to them or push them away. For example, clinging to anger may make you feel safe and self-assured but can lead to arguments with your loved ones and to stomach problems. Similarly, trying *not* to be angry, but still simmering inside, can have the same effect. The healthy alternative is to "hold" your emotions differently, in an open, aware, self-compassionate manner.

When we open to difficult emotions, we're not trying to stare them down either, making our lives miserable for the sake of peace and tranquility sometime in the future. In this chapter, you'll learn to build a balanced relationship with emotions, here and now, day by day.

HOW WE CREATE SUFFERING

We're in a better position to do something about disturbing emotions when we know how they emerge from barely perceptible origins. We can nip them in the bud. Here's a story from my own marriage.

I was looking forward to welcoming my wife home from the hospital where she had hip surgery. I wanted to show my love for her at this critical time, especially because I know that she's not the type of person who relishes being dependent on others. "This is a unique opportunity to take good care of her," I thought.

My wife is a morning person and I'm not, but I decided to get up early on her first day home from the hospital. As I arranged my wife's rehabilitation equipment—gripper, pressure sock sleeve, special shoes—I noticed I was feeling tense and grumpy. I suffer from morning hypoglycemia and had forgotten to drink some juice first thing out of bed. I decided to continue on because I wanted to be a good partner, at least for the next hour, and hid my tension by keeping silent. My wife noticed my puckered face, and an instant later I could see her become sad. "How did she pick up on my mood?" I first thought, "Was I not gentle enough while pulling on her socks?"

I felt ashamed for disappointing my wife, and started questioning my capacity to care for her. "What will happen when we're old and frail?" I asked himself. At the same time, my wife was starting to worry that she might be too demanding, yet she desperately wanted to master her rehabilitation equipment on this first morning, so she could be more independent.

As I criticized myself ("I'm probably not a caregiving person"), I felt the impulse to blame my wife for needing help so early in the morning. "She should *know* I'm not a morning person," I thought. "But, then again, how can I blame her on this very first day back from the hospital? Today is about *her* needs, damn it, not mine! Maybe we'll be done in a few minutes." We weren't.

Eventually a moment of mindful awareness dawned on me as I struggled to put her shoes on her swollen feet. "Wow, this situation is going downhill fast," I heard in my mind, "definitely not how you imagined the first morning back from the hospital. What a mess we're in!"

With that, I took a deep breath and intentionally said a compassionate statement of intent to myself, "May she and I be free from suffering," and I told my wife I needed to get a glass of orange juice. When I returned, I felt much better and resumed my efforts.

What happened here? Notice how my discomfort escalated from (1) simple sensation to (2) aversion, (3) strong emotion, (4) *entanglement* in the emotion, (5) almost taking regrettable action. Each step along the way, from the bottom up, fighting the feeling amplified the problem.

Low blood sugar initially made me feel tense (sensation). I didn't want to feel that way (aversion) on this special morning, so I tried to ignore it, which led to feeling aggravated (strong emotion). My wife felt sad when she saw that she was bothering me, which, in turn, made me feel ashamed (even stronger emotion). I got caught up in shame (entanglement) and began criticizing myself ("I'm probably not a caregiving person"), and almost in the same moment I found fault with my wife. I narrowly averted behaving badly (action)—saying something. A moment of mindful awareness—noticing how bad I was feeling—was the key to interrupting this out-of-control spiral. The entire sequence happened in a matter of minutes.

There's usually a sequence of internal events when we find ourselves very upset. A thoughtful patient of mine said this is how his mind works when he gets depressed:

- "I *don't like* this feeling."
- "I *wish* I didn't have this feeling."
- "I *shouldn't* have this feeling."
- "I'm *wrong* to have this feeling."
- "I'm *bad!*"

Emotions just seem to get stronger the more we fight them, often culminating in self-condemnation—"I'm bad!"

The earlier we interrupt the chain of negative associations, the better. If we catch our emotions "upstream," where aversion first springs out of an unpleasant sensation, we can stay calm and centered. After we're swept downstream, where strong emotions are swirling around, we still have a chance to disentangle from our suffering, but it's not so easy.

ANCHORING EMOTIONS IN THE BODY

You can see from the vignette above that emotions are part mind and part body; the body affects how we think, and thinking affects the body. Emotions always express themselves in the body. If we can identify the bodily component of a difficult emotion—tension, trembling—we can avoid getting caught up in unnecessary mental anguish. (A neurological explanation for this process is given in the following chapter.) Even intense emotions can be scaled back through body awareness.

Do We Have Free Will?

In 1999, Benjamin Libet asked participants in a brain study to randomly flick their fingers or wrists as he measured their brains' "readiness potential." He made the surprising observation that the brain became active 550 milliseconds *before* any muscles moved. It took his human subjects another 350–400 milliseconds to become *aware* of their intention to act, with about 200 milliseconds left before the finger or wrist actually moved. Our brains seem to know what we're going to do before we do! From a neurological perspective, free will is an illusion, but we still have "veto power" over an impending action if we become aware of it early enough.

Take the example of grief. When people experience grief, they're likely to have a feeling of tension or hollowness in the chest region, while at the same time thinking that they would rather not go on living without their loved one. It's much easier to manage the physical side of grief—muscle tension in the chest region—than the mental side. That's because when we think about thinking, we become absorbed in it, often adding an extra measure of self-judgment. If we locate the emotion in the body and soften into it, we can start to liberate ourselves from the mental preoccupations that characterize strong emotions like grief.

When a patient of mine is overwhelmed with emotion, we typically explore together where the feeling is located in the body. It's different for every person, but anger is often felt as tension in the neck, sadness as tightness in the chest, and shame as an empty feeling in the upper body and head. Many emotions, especially fear, are felt in the abdomen; that's why they're called "gut feelings."

It's easy to be mindful of the body because the body is slow-moving and tangible. Mindfulness of emotions is a little more difficult than mindfulness of the body, and mindfulness of thoughts is more difficult still. When we find our emotions in the body, they become anchored and can't toss us around so much. The following exercise will help you do that. It builds on the mindfulness practices you have already learned.

TRY THIS: Mindfulness of Emotion in the Body

This exercise takes 10 minutes and is best practiced when you're having a difficult emotion. If you're feeling content, pick an emotion that generally bothers you, such as anger, fear, or guilt. The first time you do this exercise, choose a *mildly* difficult emotion. Start by finding a comfortable position, close your eyes, and take three relaxing breaths.

- Note your posture on the chair as if you were seeing yourself from the outside. Feel your body humming with sensation. Enter into your body and into the world of sensations occurring in this very moment.

- Now bring attention to your heart region. If you wish, place your hand over your heart.

- Find your breath in the heart region and begin to practice mindfulness of breathing. Feel your chest move as you breathe. When your mind wanders, bring it back to the sensation of breathing.

- After a few minutes, release your attention to your breath and let yourself recall the difficult emotion. If you wish, remember the *situation* in which you felt the emotion.

- Now expand your awareness to your body as a whole. While you recall the emotion, scan your body for where you feel it the most. In your mind's eye, sweep your body from head to toe, stopping where you can sense a little tension or discomfort.

- Now choose a single location in your body where the feeling expresses itself most strongly. In your mind, incline gently toward that spot. Continue to breathe naturally, allowing the sensation to be there, just as it is. If you wish, place your hand over your heart as you continue to breathe. Allow the gentle, rhythmic motion of the breath to soothe your body.

- If you feel overwhelmed by an emotion, stay with your breath until you feel better and then return to the emotion.
- When your period of meditation has nearly elapsed, return to your breath for a few minutes and then gently open your eyes.

Did you notice that emotion could be felt in more places in your body than you originally expected? Could you sense how the body resists uncomfortable emotions? Did your body start to let go as you brought nonjudgmental awareness to the places of tension? You can practice this exercise any time you have a difficult emotion. When an emotion is released in the body, the mind lets go as well.

Sometimes it helps to *label* the feeling tone in your body. For example, you can say "unpleasant," "pleasant," or "neutral" as you sweep through the sensations in your body. Or when you feel an unpleasant sensation, you can just say "Ouch!" The idea of labeling is to be *with* the sensations without being swallowed up in them.

The following exercise can be added to the one you just did. It may help to deliberately cultivate a softer, friendlier relationship with the physical discomfort of difficult feelings.

TRY THIS: *Soften, Allow, and Love*

Again, start to practice by finding a comfortable position, close your eyes, and take three relaxing breaths.

- Bring awareness to your body and the sensations occurring there in the present moment. Then find your breath in the heart region and begin to track each breath with mindful awareness.
- After a few minutes, release your attention to your breath and let your attention be drawn to the place in your body where your difficult emotion can be felt most strongly.
- *Soften* into that location in your body. *Let* the muscles be soft without a requirement that they *be* soft, like applying heat to sore

muscles. You can say, "soft ... soft ... soft ..." quietly to yourself, to enhance the process.

- *Allow* the discomfort to be there. Abandon the wish for the feeling to disappear. Let the discomfort come and go as it pleases, like a guest in your own home. You can repeat "allow ... allow ... allow ..."

- Now bring some *love* to yourself for suffering in this way. Put your hand over your heart and breathe. You can also direct love at the part of the body that is under stress. It may help to think of your body as if it were the body of a beloved child. You can repeat "love ... love ... love ..."

- "Soften, allow, and love." "Soften, allow, and love." Use these three words like a mantra, reminding yourself to incline with tenderness toward your suffering.

- If you experience too much discomfort with an emotion, stay with your breath until you feel better.

- Slowly open your eyes when you're ready.

A soft, allowing, loving attitude toward the body is a mindful attitude. We're abandoning the instinctive tendency of the body to tense up and reject discomfort. "Softening" occurs at the physical level, "allowing" at the mental level, and "loving" at the emotional level. Together, they allow the body to release what it's holding on to. If you find one or more parts of the exercise easier, just stick with that. For example, perhaps it makes the most sense simply to "soften and allow."

"Allowing" also refers to letting *thoughts* come and go. Until now, I haven't emphasized thoughts because they're so hard to track from moment to moment. However, our thinking can have a huge impact on how we feel. How good can you feel if you're beating up on yourself, thinking "I'm an idiot" over and over? When you're aware of such self-destructive tapes in your mind (you'll learn to identify them in the next chapter), just allow them to arise and disappear in compassionate awareness.

Be careful not to work too hard at meditation or be too technical about it. The way you conduct this exercise should embody the same message that you're giving to your body. If you want to soften your muscles, do the exercise softly. If you want to allow all kinds of thoughts to slip in and out of your mind, take a back seat and watch the river flow. Let it be easy. Don't rush or harbor any expectations other than the wish to be a loving companion to yourself. Kind wishes are therapeutic in their own right even if what you're feeling is difficult.

THE ART OF LABELING EMOTIONS

You've probably seen by now how labeling sensations can keep you grounded in your body and out of your ruminating mind. Now we'll advance to labeling *specific* emotions. This practice helps you see emotions as "just emotions" rather than getting caught up in them.

In the last chapter, I gave you an instruction during the "mindfulness of sound" exercise to relinquish the tendency to label. That might seem to contradict what this chapter is emphasizing. The difference is that when the object of awareness is *neutral,* like most sounds, labeling can separate us from the experience of just sound. But when something's troubling us, the act of labeling helps us step back just enough to remain in relationship to the feeling without drowning in it. Naming emotions—"loneliness," "sadness," "fear," "confusion"—makes it easier for us to be with difficult emotions.

Noting

"Noting" is an umbrella term for *turning toward* an inner experience with awareness. We can note by wordlessly "noticing" a sensation, thought, or feeling for a second or two ("Ah-ha," "Oh yes"), or by "labeling" it with a word.

We can also ignore or *turn away* from difficult inner experience, returning to our chosen anchor, such as the breath. This is sometimes a good idea. Focusing on one object to the exclusion of others brings calmness of mind, at least for the time being. It's worth learning to "note," however, since we'll eventually have to deal with our difficult emotions, such as fear. Noting helps us do it safely: "That's fear! Yes, but it's *only* fear." I had a patient who said, "Anchoring is like 'home base,' and noting is like 'traveling.'"

In actual practice, noting *alternates* with anchoring, switching back and forth every few seconds. Don't stray from the body (your breath or another anchor) for very long. The more we allow our attention to dwell on an emotion rather than the anchor, the more we'll learn about it, but we risk losing calmness and stability of mind. Noting plus anchoring helps you maintain even, balanced attention while you explore difficult emotions.

Labeling requires more engagement with negative emotions than noticing does. It means giving a specific title to what you're going through. It draws us further into the experience, but it can also provide distance and perspective. When a strong emotion arises, you can label it out loud or move your lips quietly to mouth "anger," "anger," "anger." When an emotion is mild, you can name it silently in your mind for the same effect.

There are many ways to label our experience. One of the most common forms, when you're relatively free of emotional conflict, is simply to say "thinking" when you're entangled in thought and then return to the anchor. You can also do the same with "sensing" and "feeling." You can use the labels "pleasant," "unpleasant," and "neutral" to describe how you feel, softening the grip of attraction and aversion. You can also say, "This hurts," "Ouch!," or "disturbing" when you have vague, unspecified discomfort. We're not trying to *stop* suffering; we want to *know* when we're suffering, which loosens it up a bit. Labeling apostrophizes emotions.

Just about any inner experience can be labeled. I had a client, Luis, with attention deficit disorder who said that his main problem was "beating up on myself." He had internalized all the criticism he had received as a child for not completing his homework assignments and for being restless most of the time. Luis resolved to name self-criticism every time it occurred, both in formal and informal meditation. I asked, "How do you know when you're beating up on yourself?" Luis said, "I feel tension in my stomach, anxiety in my chest, or I find I'm short with the kids. Then I assume I'm doing it, so I say 'beating up on myself.'" This simple labeling practice gave Luis relief from self-critical thoughts.

How we label is important too. We can apply "worried attention" or "calm attention." Worried attention leads to fearful withdrawal, and calm attention gives us a little space to look around. It's like being a kid scared in the dark. Saying to yourself "It's dark and hard to see" is labeling with calm attention; it keeps you from succumbing to abject fear, exaggerating the danger with your own mental interpretations, or blaming yourself for being "a big baby." Worried attention might sound like "OH NO, I can't see a THING! Who knows what's out there?" and sets off a cascade of thoughts that turns uneasiness into terror.

Try to adopt a *gentle, accepting tone* with your labels. If you find yourself barking at an emotion, you probably have an underlying agenda of making the emotion go away, which runs counter to everything we're doing. Soft, gentle labeling helps the mind escape the tendency to wish away unpleasant experience. Also, don't work too hard at this or your attention is likely to wrap around and hold onto an uncomfortable emotion rather than release it. Go slow and easy.

Words for Feelings

Labeling emotions is a powerful way to manage them and to behave skillfully in relationships. It helps us stay calm so we can make rational decisions. Parents tell their young children to "use your words" when the child is upset. Mental health clinics hold classes for "alexithymic" adults—people who don't have words for feelings. For example, if a man cannot say "I feel ashamed," he's more likely to get angry and behave irrationally. If you think about it, the ability to find accurate labels for feelings underlies the entire "talk therapy" industry. Brain research has revealed that finding words for feelings *de*activates the part of the brain that initiates a stress response.

Labeling Emotions Calms the Brain

How does mindfulness meditation actually help balance our emotions? Is there a neurological mechanism? David Creswell and his colleagues at the University of California used functional magnetic resonance imaging (fMRI) to explore how the practice of labeling emotions calms the brain. Thirty participants were shown photographs of people who were emotionally upset, and the participants were asked to label the emotion (for example, "angry" or "fearful"). In a control condition, the participants looked at faces and selected a name underneath them that corresponded to the person's gender, like Harry or Sally. The researchers discovered that the amygdala—the part of the brain that sounds an alarm in times of danger—was *less* active when an emotion label was attached to the upset face compared to when a name was attached. Parts of the prefrontal cortex, especially the midline (the "medial" part that is active when we monitor our own emotional starts), became *more* active as the amygdala became *less* active, demonstrating that the prefrontal cortex inhibited the activity in the amygdala.

The participants were also asked to fill out a mindfulness scale. The inverse relationship between prefrontal cortex activity and the amygdala was *greater* for highly mindful participants than for those who were less mindful. (It is unclear whether the activated part of the prefrontal cortex is in or outside the default network. More research is needed to define the default network and separate out the functions of the different parts of the medial prefrontal cortex.) Creswell's research suggests a neurological "mechanism of action" for why we feel better when we talk to a friend, write in a journal, or otherwise put our feelings into words.

The best words for emotions are often quirky little expressions that may carry personal meaning. For example, if I'm feeling agitated, I might label it "squirrelly" after the little rodent that runs around making jerky movements while it gathers and hides nuts. Some people like the Yiddish expression *ferklemt* for the lump-in-the-throat feeling, or "going nuclear" for murderous rage. The longer you practice, the more nuanced, perhaps even poetic, you'll find your use of emotion words becomes.

Psychologists over the past 100 years have attempted to identify which human emotions appear to be more basic than others. There does not appear, however, to be any psychologically or biologically compelling reason to select one set of basic emotions over any other (for example, fear, love, rage; happiness, sadness; or love, joy, surprise, anger, sadness, fear). For our purposes, what matters is the *function* of the word—how well it captures a feeling and opens a little space around it.

The most comprehensive list of emotion words I've found in the English language has been compiled by linguist and computer engineer Steven J. DeRose, who organized more than 800 words into categories for easy reference. DeRose prefers to use adjectives or verbs for labeling emotions ("afraid," "boiling") rather than nouns ("fear," "frustration") because they describe the felt-sense of the emotion. Also, a word ending in *-ing* is more "ongoing in the present moment" than a word ending in *-ed*, such as "worrying" versus "worried." Sometimes, however, a person may wish to have a little *more* distance from an emotion—not feel it so much as it's happening—so you should decide for yourself which word is most appropriate for each situation. (DeRose's complete list of emotion words can be found in Appendix A.)

Although the focus of this book is on dealing with *negative* emotions, it helps to name *all* our emotions, including positive ones. That's because our positive emotions are subject to change, and when they do change, they often morph into negative emotions. For example, we feel disappointment when the infatuation phase of a new relationship wears off after 4–6 months. If we can label positive emotions, we'll hold them more lightly, just like labeling negative emotions. That protects us from disappointment when our emotions change.

It's important to remember that emotions are not inherently negative or positive. Rather, they become negative, and ultimately destructive, the more we struggle to make them go away. The formula for suffering given in Chapter 1 (Pain × Resistance = Suffering) can be restated as

Difficult Emotions × Resistance = Destructive Emotions

You'll discover that so-called negative emotions—anger, fear, hatred—are not so bad when they don't get under your skin. Instead, we can greet them (and ourselves) with mindfulness and compassion. More will be said about positive and negative emotions in Chapter 5.

Meditating on Emotions

Some of the more intense negative emotions—ashamed, enraged, despairing, numb, forsaken, repulsed, terrorized—can be difficult to identify because they can swallow us up. For example, when we feel "shame" ("I am bad"), it's as if the person witnessing the emotion has evaporated and there is no one left to do the labeling. Over time, we can get a handle on shame by recognizing how it feels in the body and by giving it a name. When we roll the word around on the tongue a few times—"shame," "shame," "shame"—it gets easier and easier to label and the emotion becomes workable.

The same is true for a powerful emotion like "hatred." Consider the following example:

Caroline was the mother of two daughters, 4 and 5 years old. Her own mother had been very patient and didn't show Caroline much irritation throughout her childhood years. Caroline had a different temperament: she was an ambitious history professor, and she excelled at sports. She felt most at ease when she was moving around, and she became cranky when things didn't go as planned.

Caroline's partner suggested she have a few therapy sessions of her own to deal with her increasing irritation with their older daughter, Emma. Caroline confided to me in therapy that she just couldn't bear hearing Emma say "I hate you, Mommy" one more time, especially when Emma didn't cooperate during meals and bath time. Her partner had no trouble with Emma. Caroline found herself resenting Emma and ignoring her in favor of her more cooperative sibling.

Caroline's role model for motherhood was her own mother, who never seemed to experience what Caroline was feeling. Between sobs, Caroline shared her darkest secret: "Sometimes I just *hate* Emma and wish she would go away!" It was all too much for Caroline—she couldn't bear her helplessness and hatred toward someone she wanted to love, and she wondered what kind of person would feel as she did.

I reminded Caroline, a history of medicine scholar, of a famous psychiatrist, D. W. Winnicott, who wrote an article in 1951 titled "Hate in the Countertransference." Winnicott wrote how caregivers, including mothers and psychoanalysts, put aside their own needs in order to minister to others who are needy and self-absorbed. This naturally creates some resentment, even hatred. Problems arise when hatred is considered unacceptable—even shameful—and drives a wedge between the helper and those she wants to help.

Caroline took this message to heart and went home, ready to allow herself to feel the hatred more openly when it arose with Emma. To her amazement, Caroline started liking Emma more and Emma started behaving better. When I saw Caroline again, she said that her hatred jumped around from one child to the other, depending on who was giving her a hard time at the moment, but she didn't get hung up on it and she was having fun with Emma again.

Caroline was simply using the power of labeling her emotions with an accepting attitude. It was a shock to Caroline's self-esteem to discover that she hated her own child, but when she realized that all mothers feel that way from time to time, she could relax and enjoy her child again. First she needed to find the word for how she felt, and then she needed to accept it.

The following mindfulness practice is a way of training yourself to recognize and label emotions:

TRY THIS: *Labeling Emotions*

This meditation takes 20 minutes. Find a comfortable, quiet place and sit in a dignified posture, relaxed but upright. Close your eyes or leave them partially open. Take a few deep breaths to relax your body.

- Bring your awareness to your body by noticing your posture and the world of sensation occurring within the body.

- Place your hand on your heart and begin mindful awareness of your breathing. Breathe through your heart. Do this for 5 minutes. Whenever you wish, you can let your hand slowly fall into your lap.

- Now release the breath, keeping your attention in the heart region, and ask yourself, "What am I feeling?" Let your attention be drawn to the *strongest* emotion in your body, even if it's only a whisper of a feeling. Use your body like an antenna.

- Give your strongest feeling a name. If you sat down for this exercise without any strong emotions percolating, you might be feeling "contentment." Perhaps you're just "curious." Eventually you'll probably find another emotion, such as "longing," "sadness," "worry," "urgency," "loneliness," "pride," "joy," "lust," or "envy."

- Repeat the label two or three times, *in a kind, gentle voice,* and then return to your breath.

- Go back and forth between your breath and your emotions in a relaxed way. Let your attention be drawn from your breath by an emotion, label it, and then return to your breath. There is no need to find an emotion if there isn't one. Then just be open to the possibility of emotions as you breathe. If you feel overwhelmed by an emotion, stay with your breath until you feel better.

- When about 20 minutes have elapsed, gently open your eyes.

Our inner life can become extremely interesting if we practice mindfulness meditation like this. If you ever become bored during this exercise, label it "bored." Boredom always changes to something else when we linger with it long enough, without prejudice. There's often an unpleasant or unfamiliar feeling lurking in the shadows just behind boredom. The practice of labeling emotions can transform us into poets, searching for subtle nuances in emotional experience, unflinching in the face of discomfort.

The more accurately we label an emotion, the more effectively we become "unstuck" from it. But please don't obsess over finding the perfect label; don't think too much about it. Choose a "good enough" label and return to the breath. Any label will suffice to keep your awareness in the present moment. Perhaps a more accurate label will occur to you later on. If not, don't worry. Let the practice be easy and take your time.

Also, don't feel the need to catalog every emotion that comes your way, like a botanist on a 1-day outing to an exotic nature park. In 20 minutes of meditation, you may have no more than three or four emotions, so leave it at that and label those particular emotions whenever they arise. For example, if I'm impatient while meditating and I'd rather be doing something else, I might say "impatience" or "urgency" whenever the feeling arises—whatever captures the felt-sense of the emotion—and then return to my breath. If I doubt that I'm doing the exercise correctly, I might say "doubting . . . doubting . . . doubting" whenever that suspicion arises. It can be interesting to find words for how you're relating to the meditation process itself, which may well be your strongest feeling at the time. The task is simply to recognize the strongest feeling happening in the present moment.

Labeling in Daily Life

Labeling in formal meditation practice is a prelude to labeling in daily life. For example, an anthropologist friend of mine was giving a PowerPoint slide presentation to a large academic audience. To his horror, a slide came up blank—every presenter's nightmare! He found himself blurting out loud, "fear . . . fear . . . fear," earning a chorus of good-hearted laughter and reversing a potential disaster.

How do we practice labeling in daily life? Follow the basic structure of the mindfulness exercises you've been doing: stop, observe, return. Whenever you're seized by a strong emotion, stop what you're doing, take a deep breath, bring your attention to your chest region, observe what feeling you're having, and name it two to three times in a gentle, loving manner. Shift your attention between your anchor and the label until the emotion loses its grip on you.

WORKING WITH TRAUMA

Opening to emotion is especially tricky for people who have suffered from trauma, such as a tragic accident or a violent crime. Over 50% of people in the United States have experienced trauma. Between 20 and 25% of women and between 5 and 10% of men were sexually abused as children. Furthermore, trauma is subjective, so it's entirely possible that the death of a loved one, a motor vehicle accident, surgery, or a divorce could have left emotional scars. That covers a lot of people.

When we sit quietly and make ourselves receptive to whatever feelings might arise, we're likely to remember traumatic events. This can be very healing if we can maintain a calm, balanced frame of mind, but it can be harmful if we become overwhelmed and reexperience the trauma as if it were happening again. Mindfulness is a way of meeting traumatic memories without getting swallowed up in them. Mindfulness is not, however, a passive activity. We still need to make intelligent decisions about how to allocate our awareness and attention.

Attention can be directed *internally* or *externally,* and it can have a *single* focus or an *open-field* focus. When we focus attention on a single object again and again, such as the breath, we become calmer. That's because we're abandoning disturbing thoughts and stopping the mind from jumping around like a monkey. When we open the field of our awareness to other thoughts and feelings, we'll inevitably discover memories and feelings that stir us up. It's helpful to learn about our inner landscape to establish a new relationship to a wide range of feelings that occur in daily life. We can become overwhelmed, however, if we don't balance open awareness with single-focus awareness—that is, return to the breath or some other anchor.

External focus is generally easier than internal focus for traumatized individuals. As our attention is drawn into the body, where trauma is stored, bad memories are more likely to surface. When attention is focused away from the body, for example, with the sound of birds singing, we will feel calmer. The *surface* of the body, such as the sense of touch, is also relatively calming compared to internal awareness.

George (in Chapter 2) wore a rubber band around his wrist that he snapped when he became engulfed in traumatic memories. He said "I want to draw a line in the sand between the past and the present, and snapping a rubber band brings me into the present." He also found that labeling his strongest emotion—"fear ... fear ... fear"—kept him from becoming entangled in the story line of his fear.

When truly overwhelmed, the best way to stabilize attention is to focus on a single *external* object, like a candle or a piece of music. If you feel comfortable moving closer to the body, then the sense of touch, like George's rubber band or his "here and now" stone, can safely ground your awareness in the present moment. Later on, you might try single focus on the breath. Once you know how to work with focused attention to regulate how you feel, you can gradually expand your field of awareness to body sensations or to labeling your emotions. Even when you're ready to explore your emotions, continue to take refuge in the anchor (breath, sound, touch) every few seconds. We're cultivating mental stability *and* emotional awareness.

If a trauma memory should arise during mindfulness practice, please don't feel the need to push through it. Timing and safety are critical. Many people with childhood trauma have a habit of gritting their teeth and doing what they think they *should* do, even if it feels bad. Always practice mindfulness with an attitude of self-kindness. Kindness is slow and patient. If you feel overwhelmed, please discontinue your practice for a while—that too is a form of self-kindness. The following chapters will explain more fully how to bring kindness to yourself when you need it the most. But please remember, if you have doubts or concerns about the practice, it's best to consult with a qualified mindfulness meditation teacher or psychotherapist.

In the last chapter and this one, you learned mindfulness of both the body and the emotions. Mindfulness is the practice of skillfully managing our attention and awareness. Attention regulation leads directly to emotion regulation. In the next chapter, we'll begin an in-depth exploration of self-compassion. Having a background in mindfulness will be a great help. Self-compassion contains all the healing properties of mindfulness practice—awareness of present experience, with acceptance—but its truly unique character comes out when dealing with intense and disturbing emotions.

4

what's self-compassion?

Before you know kindness as the deepest thing inside,
You must know sorrow as the other deepest thing.
—NAOMI SHIHAB NYE, *poet*

If you've been practicing mindfulness for a few weeks now, formally or informally, you've probably noticed more peace and contentment in your life. But you might also be feeling discouraged, thinking you don't have enough time or discipline to make it work. Especially if you're living in a tough situation, you may doubt whether this approach can help you. If so, please don't give up yet. Adding self-compassion to the mix is just what's needed when the outlook is bleak and we have only a faint whisper of hope left. Sometimes it's better when you *have* given up hope and just curiosity remains about what could happen next. If that's you, please proceed gently into the following chapters.

There are three mindfulness-based skills we can use to handle difficult emotions: (1) focused awareness, (2) open-field awareness, and (3) loving-kindness. So far, you've learned the first two. Focusing on a single object calms and stabilizes the mind, and open-field awareness helps us respond to daily challenges in an even, balanced way. Those two skills can help us see what's going on in our lives;

then, by applying loving-kindness, we "hold" our experience in a warmhearted, comfortable way.

Loving-kindness is wishing *happiness* for another person. Compassion is wishing for that person to be *free from suffering*. We can experience loving-kindness anywhere and anytime, but suffering is a prerequisite for compassion. Compassion is therefore a subset of loving-kindness.

Compassion occurs when "the heart quivers in response" to the suffering of another, giving rise to the wish to alleviate that suffering. When *we're* suffering and feel the urge to help ourselves, we're experiencing *self*-compassion.

HOW SELF-COMPASSIONATE AM I?

Mindfulness is a subject of rapidly growing interest in academic psychology. Research on self-compassion is following close on its heels. One goal of self-compassion research is to determine how it's related to other personal qualities, such as life satisfaction, coping with failure, self-esteem, and wisdom. Kristin Neff, a psychologist at the University of Texas in Austin, developed the Self-Compassion Scale that is used in most studies on self-compassion. This scale has six subscales that measure key elements of self-compassion, *self-kindness, common humanity,* and *mindfulness,* and their opposites, *self-judgment, isolation,* and *overidentification.* You can access the Self-Compassion Scale, as well as a wealth of related research, on Neff's website: *www. self-compassion.org.* You might want to take the test now to get a good measure of your current level of self-compassion, and again 1 month later, to measure the impact of your mindfulness and self-compassion practice.

Self-Kindness

Self-kindness is the opposite of self-judgment. For example, the statement "I'm tolerant of my own flaws and inadequacies" in the Self-Compassion Scale is the opposite of "When I see aspects of myself I don't like, I get down on myself." We have a tendency to judge ourselves when things don't go our way, adding insult to injury. A self-compassionate person responds to difficulties and setbacks in a warm and understanding manner rather than with harshness and criticism.

Common Humanity

When we experience misfortune, we're likely to feel we're the only person in the world who's suffering like that. We also tend to feel shame about our misfortune, as if we alone were responsible for it. Shame isolates. When our intense emotions subside and we see the situation from a wider angle, we're likely to discover that everything happens as a result of a *universe of causes* rather than exclusively due to "me" and "my mistake." All events are flowing and interconnected, at least to a small extent. Our experience is shared by others. That realization of common humanity brings relief from feeling alone and isolated.

When I'm feeling self-compassionate, I'm likely to endorse the statement on the Self-Compassion Scale that says "When I feel inadequate in some way, I try to remind myself that feelings of inadequacy are shared by most people." When I feel alone and isolated, the following is probably true: "When I'm feeling down, I tend to feel that most other people are probably happier than I am."

Mindfulness

Just as self-compassion is *implicit* in mindfulness practice, mindfulness can be found in self-compassion. Mindfulness is nonattached awareness—it gives us the ability to accept painful thoughts and feelings in an even, balanced manner. The opposite of mindfulness—overidentification—happens when we lose ourselves in emotional reactivity. Pain narrows perception. Mindful awareness helps us recognize when we're in pain, when we're criticizing ourselves, and when we're isolating ourselves and points the way out.

A mindfulness item from the Self-Compassion Scale is "When

I'm feeling down, I try to approach my feelings with curiosity and openness." The opposite of mindfulness is seen in the statement "When I'm feeling down, I tend to obsess and fixate on everything that's wrong."

IS SELF-COMPASSION NATURAL?

Although our personal experience may tell us otherwise, *self-compassion is the most natural thing in the world.* Deep within all beings is the wish to be happy and free from suffering. We're responding to this instinct when we suckle at mother's breast, when we cry from loneliness, and when we save up to buy a pink Cadillac. Everything we do, even the good feelings we derive from helping others, seems to derive from the wish to make ourselves feel better. Self-compassion practice is therefore not adding anything special to our behavioral repertoire—it's just fanning the flames of our innate desire to be safe, happy, and healthy and to live with ease, but in a more helpful way than our tendencies to grasp for short-term pleasure and to avoid pain at all cost.

First we need to recognize that we *deserve* to feel better. When we feel *really* bad, most of us engage in self-punishment rather than self-compassion. We heap on self-criticism ("This wouldn't have happened if I weren't so stupid"). We act as if suffering always points to a personal flaw rather than being a fact of the human condition. If we remind ourselves that wanting to feel better is a natural instinct, perhaps we'd be less likely to take ourselves to task when things go wrong. Wouldn't you still clean and bandage a wound when you get injured? Why not do the same for yourself when you're in emotional pain?

Actually, when bad things happen to us, we tend to have *three* unfortunate reactions: self-criticism, self-isolation, and self-absorption. Neff's three components of self-compassion direct us exactly in the opposite direction: self-kindness, recognizing the common humanity in our experience, and a balanced approach to negative emotions.

Why do we react like this? I look at it this way: the instinctive response to danger—the stress response—consists of fight, flight, or freeze. These three strategies help us survive physically, but when they're applied to our mental and emotional functioning, we get into trouble. When there's no enemy to defend against, we turn on ourselves. "Fight" becomes self-criticism, "flight" becomes self-isolation, and "freeze" becomes self-absorption, getting locked into our own thoughts.

Scientists have recently identified another instinctive response to stress—"tend and befriend." During threatening times, some people show a protective response toward offspring (tending) and seek social contact (befriending). Although the fight-or-flight and the tend and befriend responses are common to both men and women, women seem to incline more toward tending and befriending than men do. The tend and befriend response is linked to the hormone oxytocin, and the predominantly female hormone estrogen enhances the effects of oxytocin. It's therefore likely that women will feel a greater affinity for self-compassion (befriending oneself) than men do. However, since oxytocin is a buffer against the ravages of the fight-or-flight response, self-compassion is a skill worth cultivating by anyone who suffers from stress.

Another group of people who might find self-compassion unnatural or difficult to practice are those who've been neglected or abused in childhood—suffered lots of stress in the formative years. The learning process for these folks may simply take a little longer. Many traumatized people feel they don't deserve to feel good, or they haven't had much practice feeling good. Furthermore, it may be hard for them to experience emotional pain in safe doses. Painful emotions recruit earlier pains. For example, a relationship breakup can trigger a tidal wave of loneliness and shame stored up from childhood, overwhelming one's ability to focus and function.

People with early childhood trauma, however, often demonstrate remarkable compassion and kindness toward other people or specifically toward pets or young children. Most everybody seems to have someone or something toward whom they experience natural compassion. As we shall see in later chapters, if it's hard at first to feel compassion for yourself, you can use compassion for others as a vehicle to bring it to yourself.

Self-compassion can seem quite elusive at times, but since the wish to be happy and free from suffering is innate, it can't be ignored forever; some measure of success is virtually guaranteed. My own mother, who spent a lifetime raising kids and helping people in the community, has begun practicing self-compassion. She told me, at 83 years old, "I didn't know I could love *myself!*" Although my mother is one of those older people who grow softer with age, rather than judgmental and cranky, she is also the first to say that practicing self-compassion helps her take the difficulties of aging in stride.

IS SELF-COMPASSION SELFISH?

Most of us feel a little guilty when we pay attention to ourselves. "So many people have it much worse than me! My problems are nothing compared to theirs. I should just suck it up and quit complaining."

It's true that there's always someone who has it worse than you, and it's true that we should endeavor to help others whenever we can. That doesn't mean, however, that you can't take the time to care for yourself. We all require some maintenance; a little time dedicated to self-care is not a moral lapse. When we become proficient at self-compassion, a few seconds or a minute is all it takes. Comparing our troubles to those of others can also be a subtle way of denying and avoiding personal pain, which makes us hang on longer than necessary to what's bothering us.

My observation from traveling throughout the world is that people in the United States are particularly embarrassed when they feel bad. It's as if they've done something wrong—that their personality has failed them in some way. Some religious groups in the United States equate material success with being in favor with God. New Age theologies explain bad luck as bad karma, a result of previous misdeeds. These cultural factors serve to segregate and blame the victim rather than encouraging a kindly response to suffering.

Some people worry that self-compassion is a private cocoon that

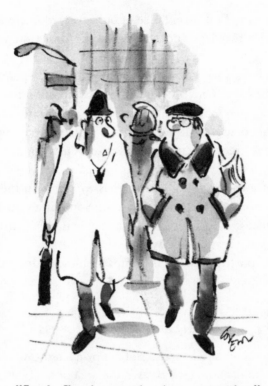

"Lately I've been getting into compassion."

will close them off from other people by making them selfish and
self-centered. The reverse is actually the case: the more openhearted
we are with ourselves, the closer we feel toward the rest of life. Self-
compassion is the *foundation* for kindness toward others. When we're
accepting of our own idiosyncrasies, we become more accepting of
others. For example, if I'm ready to criticize myself for not dressing
stylishly, I'll probably think unfavorably of poorly dressed people I
see on the street. If I feel humble and loving toward myself as I walk
out the door, in spite of my flaws, I'll greet others with a soft smile.

Accepting our flaws doesn't mean that our behavior can't or
shouldn't change for the better. *Acceptance is in the present moment.*
Each one of us has room to grow, and grow we must. We start by
befriending who we are *today,* no matter how fumbling, incomplete,

or clueless we are. Full acceptance of ourselves, moment to moment, makes it easier to adapt and change in the direction we'd like to go.

Do you have a right to this kind of radical acceptance of yourself? As you'll see when you practice self-compassion in a deliberate, conscious way (see Chapter 6), sometimes every fiber of your body tells you that focusing on yourself is a violation of a fundamental moral code. A creepy feeling comes up, even without words. This aversion may lessen when you're in great pain, but the depth of cultural resistance to caring for ourselves is worthy of mindful, that is, curious and nonreactive, introspection. Sometimes an intellectual override is necessary: "There are four people in this family; if I don't focus on myself occasionally, who will?!"

Some people think that self-compassion means indulging in self-

Empathy and Self-Awareness

Empathy for others and awareness of our own internal states seems to have a common neurological basis in the area of the brain called the *insula*. The insula is about the size of a prune and is hidden deep within the sides of the cerebral cortex. Hugo Critchley at the University of Sussex in England found that people high in empathy had more gray matter in the frontal part of the right insula. He also found that people who scored high on an empathy scale were good at tracking their own heartbeats—knowing what was going on inside their bodies. The insula seems to bring sensations into awareness, and that awareness can be used to be empathic in social interactions.

Arthur Craig of the Barrow Neurological Institute in Phoenix, Arizona, postulates that body sensations enter the rear part of the insula and are turned into social emotions—trust, contempt, guilt, pride—in the front of the insula. Thus, the insula is the "middleman" between our sensations and our emotions, the link between the body and the mind. Modulating the insula through meditation is one possible explanation for how mindful awareness of body sensations can disentangle us from troublesome emotions, as mentioned in Chapter 3.

pity. The early stages of self-compassion may indeed include pity. There's nothing wrong with that. I enjoy the line from Bob Dylan's song "Thunder on the Mountain": "For the love of God, have pity on yourself!" Self-pity, however, seems to contract our world around us, cutting us off from others, whereas self-compassion opens us to the universality of suffering among living beings. Self-compassion also has a balanced, mindful feeling to it, neither optimistic nor pessimistic. If you're sick, for example, self-compassion doesn't mean catastrophizing about the outcome of your illness. Instead, it means just being sick with a loving attitude.

Finally, self-compassion is not selfish because it's not entirely personal. In a roomful of people, it makes sense to help the person who's suffering the most, the one we know best, the one we're most capable of helping. Sometimes that person is you; sometimes it's another person. To use an airplane analogy, when cabin air pressure drops, we need to put the oxygen mask on ourselves first.

MINDFULNESS AND SELF-COMPASSION

Self-compassion practice is a special method for whittling away our stubborn tendencies to resist pain and grasp for pleasure. It's mindfulness from the neck down, emphasizing qualities of heart—motivation and emotion—rather than awareness and wisdom. The common healing element in both mindfulness and self-compassion is a gradual shift toward friendship with emotional pain. Mindfulness says, "Feel the pain" and self-compassion says, "*Cherish yourself* in the midst of the pain"; two ways of embracing our lives more wholeheartedly.

Mindfulness can lead to self-compassion, bringing in feelings of sympathy, forgiveness, tenderness, and love. In order to open our hearts, first we need to open our eyes.

I've visited India many times because I greatly admire its ancient culture, gentle people, and rich tradition of meditation. What I do *not* appreciate is the begging. Some beggars have truly heart-wrenching problems, like the man I once saw whose nose had rotted away from leprosy. Many beggars, however, are small-time opportunists. Beggars in India always cause me distress, either because of their sad condition or because of the resentment I feel when they manipulate tourists. I'm repeatedly in a quandary: Should I give a few coins? If so, am I supporting fraudulence? If not, am I selfish?

After a number of years of this distress, I recognized how much *I* was struggling whenever I encountered a beggar. I began saying to myself, "There's a beggar; here comes tension and confusion." When I focused in an accepting way on my own body, it relaxed a bit. To my surprise, I found I could meet the eyes of a beggar with a genuine smile. Occasionally I gave money and sometimes I didn't, but it always felt better than to hold my breath and avert my gaze. For some beggars, receiving a smile seemed to be even more valuable than a few coins.

Mindful awareness helped me to see beggars—those in need and those who weren't—as ordinary people trying to eke out a living. I stopped judging myself for naively giving money to a false beggar, and my heart stayed open to the truly needy. Awareness of my internal reactions opened the space for me to experience both self-compassion *and* compassion for others.

Mindfulness practice often leads to self-compassion. For example, in a research study of psychotherapists who participated in Kabat-Zinn's 8-week mindfulness training program (mindfulness-based stress reduction), significant increases in self-compassion were found after training. But we don't need to wait for self-compassion to dawn on its own in mindfulness practice. When we're in intense emotional pain and need a helping hand, we can make the implicit quality of compassion *explicit*—we can directly deliver kindness to ourselves. The following chapters will show you how to add self-compassion to the practice of mindfulness meditation.

How much self-compassion we integrate into mindfulness practice varies from person to person and from time to time. I've known long-term mindfulness practitioners who discovered the power of self-compassion only after decades of practice, having formerly disparaged it as "less rigorous." I know other people who do mindfulness meditation only after they saturate themselves with self-kindness and dedicate their practice to the benefit of all beings. In my own case, I started meditating back in the mid-1970s, spent many years practicing loving-kindness toward *others,* and now I practice a blend of mindfulness and compassion with greater emphasis on the compassion side, focusing on compassion for *both* myself and others.

During meditation, it's sometimes a relief to work exclusively with focused and open-field awareness, without the loving-kindness element. When we're in emotional turmoil, knowing how to use attention to *disregard* disturbing feelings can be a great asset—return to the breath again and again, no matter what we may be feeling. People who've experienced trauma are glad to know that they can direct their attention to safe places, externally or internally.

Sometimes we're too upset, though, to regulate our attention or even to *find* the breath. Then what? We may feel so bad that being in our own skin is like lying on a bed of nails. In times like these, recognizing our agony is the first and a crucial step toward bringing some kindness to ourselves. The next chapter reviews how to bring care and kindness to ourselves physically, mentally, emotionally, relationally, and spiritually.

Self-compassion works more with *motivation* than with attention. It's *good will* toward ourselves. Self-compassion soothes the mind like a loving friend who's willing to listen to our difficulties without giving advice, until we can sort our problems out for ourselves. We don't need to be particularly adept at regulating our attention to get benefit from self-compassion practice. We just need to know we're hurting.

The metaphor of a gracious host captures the exquisite blend of loving-kindness and mindfulness that is self-compassion. Consider the following poem by the 13th-century Persian poet Rumi:

> This being human is a guest house
> Every morning a new arrival
> A joy, a depression, a meanness
> Some momentary awareness
> Comes as an unexpected visitor

Welcome and entertain them all!
Even if they're a crowd of sorrows
Who violently sweep your house
Empty of its furniture
Still treat each guest honorably
He may be cleaning you out
For some new delight!

The dark thought, the shame, the malice
Meet them at the door laughing
And invite them in
Be grateful for whoever comes
Because each has been sent
As a guide from the beyond.

"Welcome and entertain them all!" Good will creates space for
all feelings, good and bad. We're not favoring one emotion over
another—pushing away some feelings, sugarcoating others. Just as a
gracious hostess can send her guests home feeling happier than when
they arrived, good will has a tendency to shape our feelings for the
better.

TENDING TO THE "SELF"

Perhaps the most significant contribution of self-compassion to
mindfulness practice is the attention given to the "self." When our
suffering is great, we become engulfed in the experience and identify with it. The "self" suffers. We need to shift the object of our
acceptance from the feelings we're hosting—"a joy, a depression, a
meanness"—to the host, as Linda did.

Linda had just received a diagnosis of breast cancer. Remarkably, she was not particularly afraid of dying, nor did she worry
much about the possibility of surgery. A single mom, she worried
only that her 19-year-old daughter might have to go through life
without a parent. Linda could hardly bear the thought, yet she was
preoccupied by it. She was afraid for her daughter. When Linda was

able to recognize how much *she* suffered whenever these thoughts passed through her mind, she could exhale and relax a little bit. Simply noticing her stress level helped her start to let go of her fears. Linda began to think creatively about how to prepare her daughter for the worst. Perhaps her daughter's favorite aunt would take her in? Perhaps her daughter would find a partner of her own before the worst happened?

Keeping ourselves in the picture in the midst of emotional chaos is the first step toward finding a solution. This is not easy to do. When we're in the grip of strong emotions, our attention narrows to what's in front of our noses, not what's behind them: *"That's* a problem." *"He's* a pain." We're unable to give ourselves the loving attention we need.

When couples are in conflict, for example, each person becomes absorbed in the struggle to be seen by the other. Relational conflict often comes down to "Look at me, look at me!" Each partner seeks validation for how much pain the other person has caused. This is a fruitless quest because when we start accusing one another, it's unlikely we'll ever get recognition. A better option is to redirect our attention and compassionately respond to our *own* suffering first, and then listen to our partner's suffering.

Our Personal Vulnerabilities

Each of us has personal vulnerabilities that flare up when times are tough. When we don't recognize our tender spots, they may wreak havoc in our lives. For example, if I lose my job and unconsciously think I'm a "failure," coping with being a "failure" may become a bigger challenge than finding a new job.

Self-compassion is most effective when the underlying issues associated with emotional pain are acknowledged. And it's not always easy to recognize our vulnerable areas, especially in the heat of the moment. The psychologist Jeffrey Young of Columbia University has done some of the legwork for us by identifying 18 personal "schemas"—intertwined bundles of intense emotion, body sensations, thoughts, and behaviors—that usually can be traced back to early childhood. Some schemas lead with *behavior,* perhaps a tendency to be controlling or inhibited, and others lead with *feeling,* such as mistrust or fear of abandonment. When we recognize the schemas we're dealing with, they start to lose their grip. Tara Bennett-Goleman wrote a fine book, *Emotional Alchemy,* about working mindfully and compassionately with our schemas.

If you'd like to take an inventory of your schemas, please go to *www.schematherapy.com* and order the Young Schema Questionnaire (YSQ). Otherwise, see if you can identify your vulnerable areas from the list below.

TRY THIS: *My Schemas*

Please review the following schemas and identify the ones that relate to you most closely. Sometimes two or three schemas exist together.

1. *Abandonment/Instability:* My close relationships will end because people are unstable and unpredictable.

2. *Mistrust/Abuse:* I expect to get hurt or be taken advantage of by others.

3. *Emotional Deprivation:* I can't seem to get what I need from others, like understanding, support, and attention.

4. *Defectiveness/Shame:* I'm defective, bad, or inferior in some way that makes me unlovable.

5. *Social Isolation/Alienation:* I'm basically alone in this world and different from others.

6. *Dependence/Incompetence:* I'm not capable of taking care of myself without help on simple tasks and decisions.

7. *Vulnerability to Harm and Illness:* Danger is lurking around every corner, and I can't prevent these things from happening.

8. *Enmeshment/Undeveloped Self:* I feel empty and lost without guidance from others, especially from people like my parents.

9. *Failure:* I'm fundamentally inadequate (stupid, inept) compared to my peers and will inevitably fail.

10. *Entitlement/Self-Centeredness:* I deserve whatever I can get, even if it bothers others.

11. *Insufficient Self-Control/Self-Discipline:* I have a hard time tolerating even small frustrations, which makes me act up or shut down.

12. *Subjugation:* I tend to suppress my needs and emotions because of how others will react.

13. *Self-Sacrifice:* I'm very sensitive to others' pain and tend to hide my own needs so that I'm not a bother.

14. *Approval-Seeking/Recognition-Seeking:* Getting attention and admiration are often more important than what is truly satisfying to me.

15. *Negativity/Pessimism:* I tend to focus on what will go wrong and mistakes I'll probably make.

16. *Emotional Inhibition:* I avoid showing feelings, good and bad, and I tend to take a more rational approach.

17. *Unrelenting Standards/Hypercriticalness:* I'm a perfectionist, am focused on time and efficiency, and find it hard to slow down.

18. *Punitiveness:* I tend to be angry and impatient, and I feel people should be punished for their mistakes.

You may want to select *one* schema that predominates in your life and write down a situation in which it's likely to play out. Then list (1) the *sensations* that arise in your body, (2) the *emotions* that go with the schema, (3) what you're likely to be *thinking,* and (4) how you typically *act* when the schema is engaged. (If none of the schemas given above quite fit you, make up your own.)

Here's where you can get a fix on self-destructive thinking—identify the mental themes that lead to bad feelings. For example, if your schema is "pessimism," ask yourself what you say to yourself over and over that supports your pessimism, such as "Why bother?"

and "Waste of time!" Or if your schema is "social isolation," perhaps you think, "Fine for her, but I'm different" when a great opportunity presents itself to you. It's nearly impossible to track all your thoughts in meditation, but repetitive themes are easier to recognize once we've identified them. Just observe these thoughts arise and disappear in spacious awareness.

Recognizing our schemas is mindfulness, and being kind to ourselves in the midst of an active schema is self-compassion. I've found that labeling schemas, like labeling emotions, is a remarkably effective way of managing emotions—it dissolves a whole cluster of destructive thoughts, feelings, and behaviors in one burst of kindly awareness: "Oh yes, there I go again, expecting failure!" or "There's my dependency schema again!" This practice is taught in Tara Bennett-Goleman's book.

When we understand exactly how a schema shows up in our lives, we're more likely to catch it. If I hear myself saying, "I don't know, what do *you* want to do?" because I'm afraid of making someone upset, I know I'm in "self-subjugation" mode. If I can't stop proofreading a report before I give it to my boss, I may be in the "unrelenting standards" mode. If I feel scared before I go to a party, I might be into "social undesirability." We want to *see* schemas, *feel* schemas, and then *let them go*.

Is There a Self?

Schemas are part of one's personality. We each have a unique personality—a sense of self—that feels distinct from those of others. A personality gets assembled as we grow up, and it appears to have some consistency over time. Just recall how easily you could relate to an old friend at a class reunion, as if time stood still, even if you didn't recognize him or her at first from across the room. Some things about us change, and other things stay the same.

Interestingly, most neuroscientists agree that there is no "self" to be found in the brain. In the words of Wolf Singer from the Max Planck Institute in Frankfurt, Germany, the brain is an "orchestra without a conductor." The brain is bursting with activity in all directions, but where and how a sense of separate consciousness arises from this blooming, buzzing confusion remains an open question. Additionally, through the lens of inner contemplation, a careful look at our mental activity is likely to reveal only brief moments of experience, arising and falling away. No self—only this thought, that sensation, this feeling, that impression. Even the experience of consciousness comes and goes. Who, then, am I?

A sense of "self" seems to arise spontaneously when we're in emotional pain. For example, if you're afraid to die, you might ask fundamental questions about "who" or "what" you are—*who* actually dies. When your feelings are hurt by others, you may wonder if what you're hearing is actually true. "Who am I?" The reverse is also true: when we're in "flow"—calmly, joyfully, and productively engaged—there's very little sense or care for who "I" might be.

This makes sense if you think about it. The "self" is almost always associated with the body, and our bodies are built for survival. When we're in physical danger, we fight for survival. When we're in emotional trouble, we try to defend our egos. The problem with an overly rigid sense of "self" ("I'm young, I'm smart") is that it interferes with our well-being as life changes, and the ability to adapt to changes in our lives—failure, sickness, old age—is what determines whether we'll be peaceful and happy in the long run. Trying to continually prop ourselves up against insult and injury can be very stressful.

Ironically, we need a "self" to make progress on the path of self-compassion. If there were no one around to feel the pain of a self-critical or self-isolative attitude, no change would be possible. We can cultivate a kind, gentle attitude—not rejecting, not overly prizing—toward the "self" until it no longer suffers and has no reason to assert itself.

The idea of "no-self" is a hopeful message contained in Buddhist psychology. It really means there's no *fixed* self. Even our schemas arise and disappear. The notion of "no-self" doesn't mean that we're "nobody," either. We're really part of everything. To become happier and to adapt better to changing circumstances, the task is to soften our fixed self-images and behavior patterns that reduce our freedom. Can you occasionally allow yourself to feel like a child when you're with a child, like an old man with an old man, or like a young woman with a young woman? We become everybody at one time or another, either through empathy or through the many roles and situations of our lives: young/old, bright/dull, pretty/ugly, good/bad, successful/unsuccessful. Can we let that be so, or must we cling to a favorite version of ourselves, adding an extra burden to our lives?

Ironically, the more compassion we give to the suffering "self," the more flexible it becomes. For example, if I give a lackluster speech and afterward find myself regurgitating every word in my mind, it may help to hear a loving remark such as "Well, it was just after lunch. What do you expect? Everyone would rather be napping!" Compassion from others or from within ourselves helps us accept ourselves in our discomfort. We begin to see the complexity of factors that made things go wrong, and we don't need to be the center of the universe. In the words of Simone Weil, "Compassion directed toward oneself is humility."

WHAT DOES THE RESEARCH SHOW?

Research on self-compassion is demonstrating that it softens the impact of negative events in our lives. Self-compassionate people are more likely to *recognize* when their efforts turn out badly and to take responsibility for their part. They're even more likely to recognize undesirable aspects of their own character, but they don't obsess over them so much. For example, when a self-compassionate person experiences academic failure, he or she is likely to see it as an opportunity for improvement.

Interestingly, self-compassionate people have high self-esteem, but their self-esteem is not particularly related to how others evaluate them. Self-esteem derived from self-compassion comes from how we *respond* to evaluations. Receiving a bad evaluation is an occasion for sympathy and comfort, not rumination and self-criticism. People who are self-compassionate are therefore less afraid of failure and rejection. High self-esteem seems to be correlated with narcissism, but self-compassion isn't related to narcissism. Self-compassionate people don't need to become grandiose to feel good about themselves.

Self-compassion is a relatively stable way to regulate emotions. We don't need to build ourselves up when we're feeling down, such as by using positive affirmations (for example, "Every day I'm feeling better and better about myself"). Rather, self-compassionate people enter into the truth of their experience with softness and kindness, which takes the struggle out of it.

Kristin Neff and colleagues found that self-compassion, as assessed by her scale, correlated even more strongly than scores on a mindfulness scale with measures of wisdom, personal initiative, happiness, optimism, positive affect, and coping. Self-compassion is also related to life satisfaction, emotional intelligence, and social

Dieting through Self-Compassion

A leading researcher on self-compassion, Mark Leary at Duke University, along with Claire Adams at Louisiana State University, found that self-compassion helped people avoid unhealthy foods. They gave all participants a test of "restrictive eating" that measured their desire to avoid "forbidden food" like doughnuts. The participants were then divided into different groups, and some were asked to eat a doughnut. Afterward, a bogus story was given for why they should eat a candy or *more* than one candy if they so wished. Between these activities, some participants were told, "I hope you won't be hard on yourself [for eating the doughnut]. Everyone eats unhealthily sometimes, and everyone in this study eats this stuff. ..." Highly restrictive eaters who heard this compassionate message after eating a doughnut had less distress and ate fewer candies afterward. Self-compassion appears to be a healthy way to respond to lapses in dieting. When dieters' heads are "not cluttered with unpleasant thoughts and feelings," they can focus on their dietary goals rather than trying to improve their mood by eating more food.

connectedness and inversely related to self-criticism, depression, anxiety, rumination, thought suppression, and perfectionism. It's pretty plain that self-compassion predicts psychological well-being.

Clinical scientists are now exploring whether self-compassion *training* can make important changes in people's lives. Paul Gilbert, a psychologist in the United Kingdom, developed a 12-week program of compassionate mind training (CMT) to help people suffering from high shame and self-criticism. A pilot study showed promising results. CMT works on the assumption that self-critical people have difficulty generating positive feelings through self-soothing, perhaps because they weren't comforted enough as children and didn't feel safe. Oxytocin and the opiates are activated by social affiliation and care: stroking, holding, and social support. Gilbert is currently exploring whether those neurohormones underlie the soothing effects of self-compassion training.

The research on self-compassion is currently in its infancy compared to mindfulness research, but the future of self-compassion research is promising and bright.

So far, we've learned that self-compassion is a healthy and natural response to suffering. The more we struggle emotionally, the more likely we are to be hijacked by self-criticism, self-isolation, and self-absorption. The path to emotional freedom starts with kindness toward the suffering "self." In the next chapter, we'll start to explore the many different ways we can bring self-compassion into our lives.

5

pathways to self-compassion

The time will come
When, with elation,
You will greet yourself arriving
At your own door, in your own mirror,
And will smile at the other's welcome
—DEREK WALCOTT, *poet*

The best way to understand self-compassion practice is that by doing it we're strengthening the *wish* to alleviate our own suffering. From this basic desire arise countless practical ways of taking care of ourselves. Self-compassion feels good when we practice it wisely, and the more we do, the more we want to do it. Over time a positive cycle develops, strengthening and deepening the initial motivation to practice. We just need to start somewhere.

The fact that you're alive shows that you're already taking good care of yourself. But beyond basic self-preservation, what are you doing to enhance your sense of well-being? Are you doing anything that's *not* in your best interest? How do we cultivate positive emotions—those that make us happy—without falling into old habits of resisting pain in the process? Finally, is it possible to leave our past—mental patterns that only feed suffering—behind? In this chapter we'll take a look at a wide spectrum of ways that will enable you to bring self-compassion into your life and free yourself from the clutches of unnecessary distress.

FIVE PATHWAYS TO SELF-COMPASSION

There are five key ways in which we can bring self-compassion into our lives: (1) physically, (2) mentally, (3) emotionally, (4) relationally, and (5) spiritually. Each area offers numerous practice options. Following are some preliminary ideas for how to implement them in your own life.

Softening into Your Body

How do you care for yourself *physically*? How do you relate to your body when it's under stress? A compassionate response involves softening into physical discomfort—not tightening up. Compassion is soft and tender. When the going gets tough, the *soft* get going.

Our muscles protect the body from potential danger by creating a hard shield against the world. Unfortunately, the brain doesn't easily distinguish between a threat coming from the inside and one coming from the outside, so even if you're worried about your performance on an exam, your muscles will become hard like a knot. Over time, tense muscles can put unnecessary stress on all the systems in the body.

If you're feeling tense during meditation or while sitting quietly, try softening your belly. Let it be loose and at ease. If you notice another body part that's tight, allow it to soften too. This is like the "Soften, Allow, and Love" exercise you tried in Chapter 3. With softening you're not "trying to relax," which puts pressure on you to feel something you're not. Just soften.

Do the same with your breath. When you're tense, your breath will become short and shallow. Try softening the breath a bit, perhaps by extending your belly outward as you inhale and exhale very slowly. Exhale twice as long as you inhale. Don't worry if you return to shallow breathing when you're done.

Anything you can do to soothe or comfort the body when you're under stress fits into the category of physical self-compassion. Perhaps you need to take a nap, eat nourishing food, get exercise, take a warm bath, have sex, bask in the sun, go on vacation, pet the dog, or get a massage? Allow yourself a few minutes to imagine what might help tight areas soften.

Taking care of yourself physically can also clear the mind. Are you sleeping long enough, eating properly, and getting enough exercise? There's often an inverse relationship between the mind and the body when it comes to exercise: the mind races when the body is inactive, and the mind calms down when the body starts moving.

Warm Hands, Warm Heart

In a Yale University study, Lawrence Williams and John Bargh discovered that warm hands enhance a person's emotional warmth. Forty-one undergraduates were asked to briefly hold a cup of either hot or cold coffee as they rode up an elevator with the experimenter. Afterward, in the study room, the students rated a hypothetical person on ten different personality traits. The people who had held warm coffee in their hands gave warmer ratings (generous, caring) than those who held the cold coffee.

In a second study, participants were given a bogus instruction to rate the effectiveness of a therapeutic pad—either hot or cold—that they held in their hands. As a reward for participating in the study, they were given treats they could either consume themselves or give to a friend. Those students who held and evaluated the cold pad were more likely to take the reward for themselves and those who held the hot pad were more likely to give their reward to a friend.

It appears that physical warmth is closely related to mental warmth, perhaps from associations made in childhood between physical warmth and caretaking. Recent research suggests that the insula is involved in the perception of both physical and psychological warmth. Therefore, we're likely to warm ourselves up emotionally when we drink a cup of hot tea or take a warm bath.

Some people wonder how taking antidepressant or anti-anxiety medication fits in with self-compassion practice. It's simple: ask yourself what's the most compassionate thing to do. Denying ourselves necessary medication can be a form of self-punishment or a way of ignoring our needs out of shame or obsessive concern for a "natural" body. The reverse is also true: medication can be a subtle form of emotional avoidance. Consider whether medication allows you to function better and pursue healthy behavior changes. If you feel you're ready to live without medication, please discuss it with your doctor.

The most natural way to practice self-compassion is what you're already doing. By acknowledging how we care for ourselves now, we can build on our strengths and remind ourselves of our good habits when we're under pressure. Please think in terms of *genuine* care—the kind that makes you feel truly good inside. For example, you may enjoy a cup of hot chocolate in the morning more than a cup of coffee, even though more adults drink coffee. Give

> *How do you care for yourself physically?*
>
> *Can you think of new ways to release the tension and stress that builds up in your body?*

yourself credit for knowing exactly what soothes and comforts you. Some people love to have a massage, and others would rather take a nap. How about you? Pay special attention to what you need when you're under severe stress or when things go really wrong.

Allowing Your Thoughts

How do you care for yourself *mentally*, especially when your mind is preoccupied or racing with thoughts? The compassionate response is to step back and "allow" your thoughts to come and go—to stop resisting. We want to create mental space where upsetting ideas can slip in and out of our minds naturally and easily.

What does it take to let go of unnecessary daily concerns? An ancient strategy is to use a *mantra*, which literally means "tool for the mind." You don't need a foreign-sounding word to benefit from this technique. Familiar mantras are "This too will pass" and "One day at a time." Doris Day sang the mantra *Que sera sera,* "Whatever will be will be." Repeating these phrases calms the mind, due to their meaning and the power of concentration. Whenever we return our attention to a single word or phrase, we're unhooking from our thoughts. Some people benefit by simply repeating the word "Yes" over and over in their minds. Pessimists seem to especially enjoy the mantra "If it ain't one thing, it's another!"

You can experiment with mantras that allow you to cope with different mental states. For example, a mantra that helps people stop obsessing about important decisions is "Don't know ... don't know ... don't know." A mantra for shame is "How could I have known?" A humorous mantra for the fear of disapproval is "So sue me!" Experiment with your tone of voice when you use a mantra. "So sue me" is cocky and "How could I have known?" is humble. To cultivate self-kindness, try "Be good to yourself" or "Be careful with me."

Visualizations also help us to let go of disturbing thoughts. For example, imagine your thoughts as leaves flowing down a stream, with each leaf carrying away what is on your mind. Or imagine yourself as the sky, with your thoughts as passing clouds, some dark and foreboding, some light and airy, all passing by.

A powerful strategy to hold our thoughts more lightly is to contemplate death. "How would I feel about this if I had only 1 month to live?" In the context of death, very few of our concerns seem to matter. Similarly, if we ask ourselves what we value most in life—happy kids, good health, peace of mind—we can let go of the small stuff.

> *How do you care for your mind, especially when you're under stress?*
>
> *Is there a new strategy you'd like to try to let your thoughts come and go more easily?*

Finally, when we suffer from troubling thoughts, we can cultivate compassion for our *brains*. The brain comprises only 2% of our body weight, but it works so hard that it needs 25% of our oxygen. Sometimes our overactive brains keep us awake at night simply to complete the work of the day. I know a physician who alleviated his obsessive–compulsive tendency by cultivating compassion for his overworked brain. Whenever he had an obsessive thought, he said, "Poor brain, it's happening again—so much hard unnecessary work!"

Befriending Your Feelings

How do you care for your emotional state? The compassionate way is to befriend painful emotions—to stop fighting them. There are many words for this: *empathy, concern, kindness, care, forgiveness, mercy, benevolence, thoughtfulness, tolerance, supportiveness, acceptance, understanding, friendliness, sympathy.*

Brian was a middle-aged guy who worried obsessively about his health. He went straight to the doctor whenever he felt pain. To manage his anxiety, Brian learned mindfulness meditation from a local meditation center. I taught him self-compassion techniques. After a few months of what his wife and I thought was steady progress, Brian declared to me, "You know, none of those things I've learned do me any good!"

So I asked him, "How are they not helping?" He responded, "Well, I'm just as anxious about every ache and pain, expecting it'll kill me! And my wife is getting sick of it, since I go to her for reassurance every time."

This led us to a much deeper discussion about Brian's anxiety, touching on the following important points:

- He came by his anxiety naturally, due to severe health problems in his childhood and obsessive–compulsive disorder in his family history.
- Anxiety happens in life whether we like it or not.
- Brian's favorite form of anxiety is obsessing.
- We can't argue with emotions—that will only make them worse.
- Everyone suffers in life—health anxiety is his particular hardship.

- Our therapy goal was to become more *accepting* of anxiety, not to have less anxiety per se.

- He needed to learn to hold anxiety with more kindness and less aversion.

Then Brian said, "You mean I should just let myself *feel sorry for myself?*" I replied, "Well, yes, that's a start."

Brian had a moment of "creative hopelessness," as psychologist Steven Hayes might say, and the road to recovery began with tenderness toward his own plight.

Like the sympathy Brian learned to give himself, *forgiveness* is an important aspect of emotional self-care. Many of us find it hard to forgive ourselves when we make mistakes. We extend no mercy to ourselves. One way to forgive oneself is to ask, "What would my best friend say?" Or, as the saying goes, "What would Jesus [Buddha, Krishna] say?" By taking the more benign perspective of others, we can extract ourselves from our ruminations.

Most of this book is about how to become friendlier toward uncomfortable emotions, and toward ourselves. Treating ourselves to enjoyable activities can help. Examples are:

- Listening to music
- Going on vacation
- Flying kites
- Going to church
- Thinking about sex
- Reading a novel
- Buying CDs
- Driving
- Working in the garden
- Riding a bike
- Going to the movies
- Cooking delicious food
- Collecting shells

> *How do you already care for yourself emotionally?*
>
> *Is there something new you'd like to try?*

Engaging in activities that are *intrinsically* enjoyable, rather than those that feel like work, is a way to care for ourselves emotionally.

The following two chapters will introduce a core practice for caring for ourselves emotionally—loving-kindness meditation—that you can practice anytime, night or day.

Relating to Others

Connecting with others is another form of self-care—to stop isolating. Remember that feeling connected to other human beings is a component of Neff's definition of self-compassion. We can feel isolated from others whether we are actually alone or not.

A sense of isolation can turn even ordinary unhappiness into despair or minor anxiety into dread. This is how elderly people often feel when they live alone and encounter health problems—each new symptom is a sign of imminent disaster. We may not notice when our support network is growing thin because isolation is an error of omission—it's a problem you *can't* see. Therefore, we should give special attention to our relational world.

How we relate to others has a huge impact on how we feel inside too. For example, we're unlikely to have a good night's sleep after a day of lying, stealing, and cheating. Such behavior may promote survival in the short term, but it does little for our emotional well-being. For starters, it puts us at a distance from ourselves—makes us argue with ourselves—which puts us at a distance from others.

Kindness in relationship means that our actions are guided by the wish to help others and refrain from harming them. The Dalai Lama calls this "wisely selfish" because it inspires people to be kind to us in return. The memory of a warm interaction can also give us lasting happiness.

I'm reminded of a story about a 9-year-old girl named Shanti from a well-to-do family in Mumbai, India. Shanti was walking along the beach with her father on her birthday. There are always poor people begging and doing tricks on the beach there for money. Shanti asked her father for a treat—an ice cream—since it was her birthday. Her father agreed. As they were walking toward the ice cream stand, a beggar cried out to them. Shanti then asked her father to give money to the beggar. Her father gave her a choice: spend the money on an ice cream or give it to the beggar. Shanti thought for a moment and then asked her father to help the stranger. Later that evening, as her father was putting her to bed, Shanti said sweetly, "You know, giving to the beggar was the best part of my day!" She had discovered at an early age the long-term happiness in kindness to others.

Our behavior has an impact on others—for better or worse—in many different ways. For instance, our survival depends on killing

Spending Money on Others

Elizabeth Dunn, a psychologist from the University of British Columbia in Canada, and colleagues reported in *Science* that spending money on others makes us happier than spending it on ourselves, once our basic needs are met. They explored this hypothesis in three ways: in a national survey, in a survey of people who received a profit-sharing bonus from their company, and by giving people money to spend and measuring how they felt at the end of the day.

In the survey study, 632 Americans were asked to rate their general happiness, declare their income, and identify what they spend their money on. Money spent on others (charity, gifts) was correlated with happiness, and money spent on themselves (bills, expenses, gifts to oneself) was unrelated to happiness, regardless of how much money people earned. In the study of people who had an economic windfall, employees who contributed more of their bonus to others experienced greater happiness 6–8 weeks later, and how they spent the money was a stronger predictor of their happiness than the size of the bonus itself. Finally, when people were given $5 or $20 to spend on themselves or others by 5:00 P.M. the same evening, giving away as little as $5 a day made a significant difference in how happy they felt.

and eating other living beings or plants. I knew a psychiatrist from Kansas who treated immigrants who worked at a slaughterhouse. He told me that his patients are traumatized from killing animals all day long, 5 days a week. When we eat, we usually don't think of the emotional impact that providing our food might have on the people who do it. But since we're part of the cycle of life, we should try to reduce suffering whenever we can and forgive ourselves for how we harm others, intentionally and inadvertently. We do this for our own good.

> *How or when do you relate to others that brings you genuine happiness?*
>
> *Is there any way that you'd like to enrich these connections?*

Trying to be helpful to others can become a habit and even bring happiness at the time of death. A Zen master once gave the following advice on how to die without fear: Ask the question "How can I help?" with your very last breath. Imagine having no concern for yourself in your final moments: How peaceful would you feel?

Nourishing Your Spirit

By "spirituality," we typically mean the intangible aspects of our lives: God, soul, values (love, peace, truth), or sacred connections. For most people, spiritual practice is about cultivating closeness to an ideal transcendent being, a process that, one hopes, reduces our selfish desires and personal limitations. That's a top-down approach to spirituality. Others take a bottom-up approach, where intimate contact with the miracle of daily life—the imperfect reality happening right in front of our noses—is the way. Most spiritually minded people see the need for *both* approaches in their lives: to be uplifted by a transcendent ideal and yet to remain grounded in ordinary reality.

These two approaches share a common process: taking ourselves more lightly. The "self" gets whittled away by loving God as well as through deep appreciation of the precious, fleeting nature of worldly existence. The result is that we have less "self" to protect and promote in the world. What a relief that can be, to ourselves and others. The principle behind spiritual self-care is commitment to our values—to stop "selfing."

Some people believe it's against their religion to care for themselves. Most religious traditions emphasize the importance of compassion for *others*: "Love your neighbor as yourself." But even the man who spoke those words escaped into the mountains when the crowds became too big. We read in Proverbs 11:17, "The merciful man does himself good, But the cruel man does himself harm."

What's implied in most religions is that you *already* love yourself. In the words of the Buddha:

> On traversing all directions with the mind
> One finds no one anywhere dearer than oneself
> Likewise everyone holds himself most dear,
> Hence one who loves himself should not harm another.

In fact, loving oneself is often given as an *example* of what it means to love others. It's the standard: "In the same way, husbands must love their wives as they love their own bodies. A man who loves his wife loves himself" (Ephesians 5:28).

But people feel ambivalent about themselves nowadays. It can't be assumed anymore that we love ourselves. This book was written to fill that gap. Perhaps a better example of spontaneous, unqualified love might be how we naturally feel toward a beloved pet or an innocent child. Tracking this feeling can teach us how to love ourselves better. Once we've relearned to love ourselves, we can extend it more fully to others.

Spiritual self-care usually means taking the time to cultivate the values that we hold dear. If you don't attend to your values, you'll unconsciously absorb the values of our consumer culture: pleasure-seeking, materialism. Are you regularly meeting with people who share your faith? If you

> *What do you do to care for yourself spiritually?*
>
> *If you've been neglecting your spiritual side, is there anything you'd like to remember to do?*

enjoy connecting with nature, do you get outdoors once a week? Is your religious practice nourishing you, or are you just doing it out of obligation? Are you learning to relate to yourself and others with more kindness and ease?

Just as a parent tries to attend to every aspect of a child's life—physical, mental, emotional, relational, and spiritual—we can cultivate those skills toward ourselves. If you didn't get this kind of care, or if you learned those skills and they fell into disuse after you reached adulthood, you can relearn them now. All it takes is willingness and a little creativity.

NONHARM

At its most basic level, the practice of self-compassion means not harming ourselves. It's often easier to notice when we're harming ourselves than it is to discover ways of being nicer to ourselves. Consider the following:

- How do you brush your teeth? Gently? Harshly?
- Do you rush around in the morning?
- Does your body feel tense or stiff from lack of exercise?
- Are you fatigued?
- Do you overeat?
- Do you get stuck in front of the computer?
- Do you have sex just because you feel you *should*?
- Do you resent going to so many social events?
- Do you rage at politicians on TV?
- Do you overspend on the holidays?
- Do you have to speak with your mother *every* Sunday?

The devil is in the details. Most of the harmful things we do to ourselves are unconscious habits. We don't stop and ask ourselves what we want or whether there's a good reason for it. The first question to ask when you start practicing self-compassion is "Is this harming me?" If it is, drop it. When you know how it feels to feel good, and think you deserve it, a red flag will go up when you're harming yourself and you'll probably stop what you're doing.

We also have *mental* habits, mostly unconscious, that cause us trouble. For example, if your attention is unrestrained, jumping from one thing to another, you'll suffer from mental agitation. And a perfectly good day can be spoiled if you find yourself entangled in disturbing emotions—brooding about the past or worrying about the future. An awareness practice like mindfulness meditation is a useful antidote to these common types of mental suffering.

One mental habit that can wreak havoc in our lives is *self-judgment*. If you watch your mind for 10 minutes after something goes wrong, you'll probably notice that you're criticizing yourself. It's undoubtedly useful to know what went wrong and to correct our mistakes, but usually we go way beyond that. What can we do about self-judgment? It doesn't work to "just stop judging yourself" because you're likely to judge yourself for judging yourself. (Remember, what we resist persists.) The best solution is simply to "witness" judgments, letting them come and go.

TRY THIS: *Counting Self-Judgments*

Mark out 15 minutes in the course of an ordinary day for this exercise. Choose a time when your mind might wander, maybe while you're driving a car or eating a meal alone. Say to yourself, "Over the next 15 minutes, I'll check every minute or so to see if I'm having a self-critical thought." If you have an electronic device that beeps, you can program it to ring every minute. Don't worry about remembering the *content* of your thoughts. Make a mental tally, perhaps counting on your fingers, of how many times you criticize yourself.

It's not easy to recognize self-critical thoughts because they happen so quickly. Sometimes it helps to focus on the body; if there's a little tension in your stomach, perhaps you were having a critical thought. It's okay to go back a few seconds to what you were thinking a moment before you felt physical tension. Ironically, the *intention* to be aware of self-judgment starts to eliminate the habit, even if you miss most of what's happening in your mind.

SAVORING

Savoring refers to the "capacity to attend to, appreciate, and enhance the positive experiences in one's life." It's a self-kindness to savor. The opposite of savoring is raining on your own parade. Consider the following questions:

- Do you let yourself enjoy a compliment?
- Have you lingered over a delicious meal lately?
- Can you revel in the love you feel for certain people?
- Are you prone to take a deep breath of fresh autumn air?
- Do you let yourself laugh out loud when you're happy?
- Is it okay to feel pride in accomplishment?
- Do you take pictures to remember great times?
- Do you have friends who really know how to enjoy themselves?

We shouldn't cling too tightly to positive experiences because that will cause suffering when they disappear. But we don't want to *avoid* happy moments because we're afraid of losing them either. It takes courage to savor positive experiences.

Emily Dickinson wrote:

> I can wade Grief—
> Whole Pools of it—
> I'm used to that—
> But the least push of Joy
> Breaks up my feet—
> And I tip—drunken—

Are you ready to open the door to both positive *and* negative experiences?

Savoring is a variation on mindfulness. When we savor, there's the intention to *enter fully* into the experience, rather than cling to it or drag it out. The goal of mindfulness is not to get "hooked" by positive or negative experiences—to let things be just as they are, fully and completely. In an advanced state of mind, we can savor grief and sorrow too. Research has shown that the savoring of pleas-

Interventions for Happiness

Martin Seligman, the father of positive psychology, and colleagues tested the effectiveness of five different strategies to increase happiness. Five hundred seventy-seven participants volunteered on the Internet to do an exercise for 1 week. There were six groups, including a comparison group, each with a different assignment. Two of the assignments significantly increased happiness and decreased depression. They were:

- **Using signature strengths in a new way.** Participants took an online test to learn about their top five personal strengths—"their signature strengths." Examples are "humility," "playfulness," and "love of learning." Participants were then asked to use their strengths in a new and different way every day of the week.

- **Listing three good things in life.** Participants wrote down three good things that happened to them that day and were asked to consider why they happened every night for a week.

Interestingly, the largest *initial* increase in happiness came after yet another strategy, the "gratitude visit," in which participants wrote a letter to someone who had been especially kind to them (and had not been thanked), and they delivered it. However, this emotional boost didn't last beyond 3 months. The other two techniques still had a positive effect 6 months later. Many participants continued to do their happiness interventions beyond the first week, even though they promised not to, and they were rated the happiest of all.

ant experiences can become a habit that elevates our baseline level of daily happiness.

You can also savor your own personal qualities. Enjoying what you do well doesn't mean you have to be arrogant about it. If you wish, you can take a scientifically valid inventory of your "signature strengths." Please go to *www.authentichappiness.sas.upenn.edu/Default. aspx* and click on *VIA Signature Strengths Questionnaire*. It's free of charge, and your strengths will only be ranked against one another for yourself, so you needn't be worried about what you might learn.

After you've identified your strengths, you can intentionally apply them in your daily life. For example, if you're naturally "curious," create opportunities to learn new things. If "humor" is your strength, let yourself be entertained. Also, when you're going through a tough time, remind yourself of your strengths. If "bravery" is your strength, use that special quality when you're in need. If it's "humility," find your way through with humility.

CULTIVATING POSITIVE EMOTIONS

Our emotional landscape consists of positive emotions—those that make us happy—and negative emotions—those that make us suffer. Cultivating positive emotions is therefore a compassionate thing to do for ourselves. But let's do it mindfully—not pushing negative emotions away, not clinging to positive ones. As you'll see, it's good to understand the value of positive emotions and to enjoy them.

What Are Positive Emotions?

Positive emotions have at least *two* noteworthy qualities: they feel good and they reach beyond the individual. Examples include affection, cheerfulness, zest, hope, surprise, and awe. Happy people feel connected to their environment, and unhappy people feel separated from it. Most positive emotions include regard for other people.

Compassion, for example, is an emotion that keeps us in touch with others even when it's difficult to stay connected.

Negative emotions feel bad, and they separate us from others. Examples include hatred, anger, disgust, guilt, sadness, shame, anxiety, and pity. Anger pushes people away, and sadness disconnects us if our response is to curl up within ourselves. Pity, for example, is a *slightly* less positive emotion than compassion because pity implies a feeling of separateness from the suffering individual. When we "take pity on" someone, we're moved to help, but we probably don't feel as if we're equals—on the same level.

Sadness is a "soft" emotion—there can be an opening to others, a readiness to receive help. Anger and hatred, in contrast, are "hard" emotions that flatly reject others. Soft feelings—sadness, guilt, rejection, embarrassment—require that we befriend them and go through them, feel them until they pass on their own. Hard feelings like anger require different treatment. We "let go" or "abandon" anger and hatred, whereas soft feelings become workable when we pass *through* them. When we let go of hard feelings, we usually discover soft feelings underneath. For example, beneath anger is often longing for connection, fear, sadness, or loss.

Negative emotions serve a useful function by alerting us to a problem. Our emotional or physical well-being might be in jeopardy when we feel negative emotions, and we should take heed. For example, bodyguards know that a sense of fear is a better defense against getting mugged than a black belt in karate. Fear will tell us where not to go and when to run. Likewise, sadness can alert us to a disconnection in relationship that could, left undetected, jeopardize the well-being of our families. We don't want to *eliminate* negative feelings—we just don't want to get stuck on them.

Feeding Positive Emotions

It appears that positive emotions have ample benefits. A review of over 225 published papers showed that positive emotions are related to happiness, and happy people are more likely to be successful in life and resilient in the face of misfortune. They're often more cre-

The Emotional Brain

Emotions originate in the midbrain, in the limbic system.

The limbic system developed in mammals, which needed to bond with their young, work together in groups, and communicate in elaborate ways with one another. Contrast this to the emotional displays of a crocodile, whose survival depends mainly on fear, hunger, and sex. Reptiles have rudimentary elements of the limbic system, but not enough to add emotions to instinctual urges. Humans have the most elaborate brain, including a layer of nerve cells covering the entire brain—the neocortex—that allows us to think rationally and experience consciousness.

Signals from the emotional brain are analyzed by the neocortex, which communicates back to the emotional centers. For example, the amygdala, an almond-shaped structure deep in the middle of the brain, may quickly analyze a piece of rope lying on the road as a dangerous snake. The amygdala signals the body to flee, as it also sends a message to the neocortex for further analysis. If the neocortex determines that the snake is only a rope, it communicates back to the amygdala to turn off the alarm. In this way, our rational mind can control emotional reactivity.

Human beings are not built for happiness; we're built for survival. Those of us with uncommunicative limbic systems probably did not live to see another day. The limbic system signals us to resist and avoid physical discomfort at every turn. Unfortunately, it does the same for emotional discomfort. We need a substantial intellectual override—activation of the neocortex—to teach our limbic system that resisting emotional pain is counterproductive.

This was the challenge that faced the Buddha 2,500 years ago. When he taught that resistance to pain multiplies our problems, he was trying to overcome 5 million years of human evolution. His life goal was to discover a practical psychology that would lead to freedom from suffering. Buddhist psychology and the science of mindfulness and acceptance-based psychotherapy prime the neocortex to take emotional discomfort "under advisement" rather than slavishly try to eliminate it. Neuroscientific studies by Sara Lazar, Richard Davidson, Norman Farb, and their colleagues demonstrate how mindfulness and compassion meditation can change the functioning and structure of the limbic system.

Smile Your Way to Happiness

Psychologists LeeAnne Harker and Dacher Keltner wondered whether emotional differences between people shape the outcome of their lives. They measured the intensity of smiles of 21-year-old women from their 1958 and 1960 college yearbook photographs. An intense smile had crinkled skin in the corners of the eyes, like crow's feet, and an upturned angle of the lips. Later, at ages 27, 43, and 52, the women were asked about their health and well-being. Women with intense smiles in their college yearbooks were happier at every age point. (The effect of physical attractiveness, which is related to happiness, was controlled in the data analysis.) Strong smilers were "more organized, mentally focused, and achievement oriented and less susceptible to repeated and prolonged experiences of negative affect." They were also more likely to be married by age 27 and to have satisfying marriages 30 years later.

In another surprising study, Deborah Danner and colleagues at the University of Kentucky examined autobiographies of 180 Catholic nuns, written when they were about 22 years old as they entered the convent in the late 1930s and early 1940s. Their handwritten life sketches were coded according to positive or negative emotional content. For example:

- *Sister 1 (low positive emotion):* "I was born on September 26, 1909, the eldest of seven children, five girls and two boys. ... My candidate year was spent in the Motherhouse, teaching Chemistry and Second Year Latin at Notre Dame Institute. With God's grace, I intend to do my best for our Order, for the spread of religion and for my personal sanctification."

- *Sister 2 (high positive emotion):* "God started my life off well by bestowing upon me a grace of inestimable value. ... The past year which I have spent as a candidate studying at Notre Dame College has been a very happy one. Now I look forward with eager joy to receiving the Holy Habit of Our Lady and to a life of union with Love Divine."

Sixty years later, the researchers discovered that 54% of the nuns with relatively few positive emotion sentences in their autobiographies had died, compared to 24% of those with mostly positive emotion sentences. Positive emotions in early adulthood appears to be strongly associated with longevity.

ative, less racially biased, more likely to succeed at work, and have more satisfactory relationships.

The research also shows that positive emotions allow us to see the big picture. Our vision is not narrowed by survival-based self-interest. This suggests that if we want to be mindful of whatever arises in our field of awareness, a minimum standard of happiness must exist. Meditation teachers know this: they often give love and support in personal interviews before sending students back out to meditate. Psychotherapy operates similarly—it makes a person a little happier and supplies the courage (from the French *coeur*, meaning "heart") to explore and master life's problems.

The question is how to mindfully shift the balance of emotions toward the positive. There's a story to illustrate this.

> One evening an old Cherokee told his grandson about a battle that goes on inside people. He said, "My son, the battle is between two 'wolves' inside us all.
>
> "One is Evil. It is anger, envy, jealousy, sorrow, regret, greed, arrogance, self-pity, guilt, resentment, inferiority, lies, false pride, superiority, and ego.
>
> "The other is Good. It is joy, peace, love, hope, serenity, humility, kindness, benevolence, empathy, generosity, truth, compassion, and faith."
>
> The grandson thought about it for a minute and then asked his grandfather: "Which wolf wins?"
>
> The old Cherokee simply replied, "The one you feed."

How do we feed emotions? An emotion is essentially a habit that we can either strengthen or weaken. It's not a "thing" or a "substance." For example, the hydraulic model, where anger is a reservoir of emotion waiting to be siphoned off, simply doesn't fit the data. Research shows that expressing anger actually *increases* the likelihood that we'll get angry again. The only way to reduce anger is to stop practicing it—to stop feeding the emotional habit.

So how do we unwittingly feed a negative emotion like anger? When we struggle with anger by obsessing why such-and-such happened and what we're going to do about it, we're feeding it. When we turn away in denial, but it lingers in the back of our minds, we're feeding it. When we hang on to anger because it makes us feel strong and certain, we're feeding it. In sum, resistance feeds negative emotions. They weaken if we stop regurgitating them in our minds and maintain a mindful, compassionate attitude.

And how do we feed *positive* emotions? Positive emotions naturally arise when we embrace our moment-to-moment experience fully and completely. Even anger can be transformed into something positive when we don't resist it because anger communicates important information about our world. The habit of relating to *all* our experience with mindfulness and compassion is the foundation for positive emotions (that is, emotional habits) like joy, peace, generosity, and love.

The Wisdom of Selflessness

A flexible sense of self is necessary to cultivate positive feelings. The less "self" we have to defend and protect, the more likely it is that socially positive emotions like tolerance, generosity, and acceptance will emerge. In contrast, if we identify with a fixed image of ourselves, or a particular ideology, we may feel the need to incessantly fight for our psychological survival.

Wisdom includes the direct realization of how everything changes, including ourselves. The modern Indian sage Nisagradatta Maharaj wrote:

> Love says, "I am everything."
> Wisdom says, "I am nothing."
> Between these two my life flows.

When we make the shift to seeing ourselves as transitory events—as verbs rather than as nouns—we can step back and allow the flow to continue. Our efforts shift from controlling the circumstances of our lives to learning how to meet each brief moment fully and wholeheartedly.

Selfing and the Brain

There appear to be two neurologically distinct ways of relating to personal experience: (1) moment to moment, or "experiential" and (2) as a "self," or "narrative." Norman Farb and colleagues at the University of Toronto scanned people's brains as they did tasks that evoked each of these two modes. Participants saw adjectives like "confident" and "melancholy" and were asked either (1) to sense what was going on in their body and mind or (2) to judge whether the trait applied to them.

As expected, the latter, "self"-oriented task activated brain areas associated with the "default network" and the wandering mind (see Chapter 2). Present-moment awareness, in contrast, helped participants *disengage* the medial prefrontal cortex of the default network (areas that link the past to the future and give coherence to the "self") and instead *engage* the insula and lateral brain areas (regions more closely associated with body awareness). Of particular interest is that people trained in mindfulness meditation were able to achieve this uncoupling more readily than novices. This research suggests that we can train our brains to be less preoccupied with narrative thinking—how daily events affect the "self"—and instead experience the emotional freedom of moment-to-moment awareness.

CHILDHOOD ROOTS

Is it actually possible to raise our happiness level? Aren't the emotional patterns laid down in childhood and through family genetics too strong to overcome? And how do children learn to be kind to themselves?

Can We Change?

New research by psychologist Sonja Lyubomirsky and her colleagues shows that our overall happiness level is determined by our genes, circumstances, and intentional activity. "Happy genes" account for about half of our happiness (50%). "Circumstances"—the conditions of one's childhood and present circumstances like being married, well-paid, religious, and healthy—cover a mere 10%. The most interesting category is the 40% that refers to "intentional activity"—our activities and outlook. That's what we *do,* such as exercising and spending time with friends; how we *think,* such as cultivating gratitude or kindness; and how *engaged* we are in our interests and values.

This means that, in contrast with what a lot of us believe, winning the lottery (circumstances) isn't going to make you happy for life. You'll probably return to your old happiness set point (determined by genes and the rest of your circumstances) *unless* you use the money to do what you like, like learning to play the mandolin or volunteering at your church, temple, or mosque (intentional activity). If you want to feel measurably happier, you should invest in intentional activity—how you spend your time and how you think—rather than simply acquiring a particular object or life circumstance like a BMW or a new spouse. If you do acquire a BMW or a new spouse, learn to savor those things for a long time to elevate your happiness level. Cultivating intentional activity is an antidote to the hedonic treadmill described in Chapter 1.

Learning to Relate to Ourselves

Self-compassion practice is an intentional activity, and it's closely tied to our early childhood experience. How we treat ourselves depends, in part, on how we were treated by our parents. Therefore, the circumstances of our early lives affect our ability to fully utilize the power of self-compassion.

The scientific study of how a child adapts to his or her caregivers is known as "attachment theory" and was pioneered by John Bowlby, Mary Ainsworth, and Mary Main. For example, if the primary caregiver is emotionally responsive and can "mirror" the emotions of the child ("Yes, I know you're feeling sad, dear"), the child learns what it means to be sad, angry, afraid, excited, joyful, tired, and so forth, and that it's *okay* to feel a wide range of feelings. If, in contrast, the caregiver becomes enraged whenever the child is angry, the child will push anger underground because it threatens the bond with the parent. As an adult, such a child is likely to criticize him- or herself for being angry, rather than responding to anger with self-kindness.

If the parent patiently acknowledges when the child is expressing negative emotion, the child can grow in self-awareness without danger. Such children feel secure with others. For example, a young child with secure attachment will explore a roomful of toys, and when the parent leaves the room, the child will express distress. When the parent returns, the child will initiate physical contact and return to play after he or she has settled down. These children learn to appreciate connection with others.

A child who shows no distress when the parent leaves, and seeks no contact when he or she returns, may grow up to be isolated or dismissive of relationships. A child who is unduly concerned about the parent's leaving, who can't explore his or her surroundings, and who isn't comforted when the parent returns, is likely to become an angry, passive, or fearful adult who has difficulty calming or soothing him- or herself. Such nonverbal emotional habits are transferred from childhood into adulthood.

We also *internalize* images of caregivers who mattered to us when we were young. If a girl's mother was patient and interested in her, she's likely to carry that role model inside her and relate to herself and others in the same way. Having an inconsistent or abusive parent deprives the child of knowing how to be kind to him- or herself, perhaps even of knowing that feeling good is an acceptable emotional state. I know adults who were abused as children who feel that they need to work themselves to the bone or they risk being called "lazy" or "bad." They feel like robots and resent others who work much less and still feel okay about themselves. We carry these internalized images of our caregivers, and the thoughts and behaviors attached to them, long into adulthood. A former client of mine, Andrew, is an example.

Andrew telephoned late one winter evening in despair. He was driving home from work in his truck, just after a light rain had begun to freeze on the road. As he tried to slow down for a stoplight, his truck slid straight into the car stopped before him. No one was hurt, but he crumpled the trunk of the car ahead of him. This accident happened one week after Andrew had argued successfully with his wife to raise their auto insurance deductible to $1,000. Andrew was upset, but not quite so much about the money as about the mishap.

As a little boy, Andrew had often felt unwanted. He recalls that when he went to college, his parents refused to let him come home for the holidays, falsely claiming it was too expensive. Andrew would have taken a 12-hour bus ride home from college if he had been allowed to do so.

It was an important step for Andrew to call me. When things went wrong, Andrew usually reacted with isolation and self-judgment. He was learning that these reactions were self-harming, and he didn't want to repeat them any longer. In our phone conversation, Andrew reflected on what he might have said to a friend who had a similar problem. Would he have told a friend that he was stupid to drive on the ice? *No, never!* Andrew recognized that his car problem could have happened to anyone—that it was just that, a *car* problem.

Before we hung up, Andrew recalled that he had been verbally abused whenever he inconvenienced his mother—for example, when he crashed his bicycle into a curb and bent the wheel rim. Andrew felt he was having an emotional memory and was mimicking the treatment he received as a child. Andrew vowed to respond with "compassion first" when difficulties like this happened again.

In this example, Andrew was learning how to meet his emotional habits from childhood with a new intention: self-compassion. We can learn to deal with whatever arises in the present moment even if our caregivers didn't show us how. The influence of both genetics and a difficult childhood can be softened if we relate to our moment-to-moment experience with more mindfulness and greater kindness.

You now have a broad overview of how self-compassion can be integrated into your life and why it matters. But reading about self-compassion is like scanning a recipe: it may pique your appetite, but it can't satisfy your hunger. The next two chapters will focus on the practice of loving-kindness. This is an ancient practice for developing compassion at a very deep level of your mind. You'll recognize all the mindfulness and self-compassion principles mentioned so far bundled into this one practice. Please plan to give yourself some time to actually *do* the practice—to *feel* how loving-kindness works inside your body and mind. You deserve it.

Part II

practicing
loving-kindness

caring for ourselves

I have great faith in a seed. Convince me that you have
a seed there, and I am prepared to expect wonders.
—HENRY DAVID THOREAU, *writer-naturalist*

When Henry David Thoreau wrote in the early 1860s that
he had "faith in a seed," he was challenging the popular view that many plants spring to life without seeds or
roots. As a careful observer of nature, Thoreau knew otherwise. A
keen witness of human behavior can also see that people with self-
compassion are continually planting seeds of self-kindness, nurturing the tender saplings, and weeding out unwelcome competition.

This part of the book introduces a meditation practice that has
the power to transform how you perceive and relate to your world:
loving-kindness meditation. It can be practiced intensively in formal
sitting meditation or informally throughout the day. In this chapter, you'll learn to plant seeds of loving-kindness in place of self-
criticism, self-doubt, and self-isolation. The next chapter will focus
on your relationships with others.

Loving-kindness meditation is the core practice of this book.
You may want to spend a week on this chapter alone, trying out the
practice for yourself. Pause between the sections to see if what you're
reading is true to your own experience.

A BRIEF HISTORY OF LOVING-KINDNESS

Loving-kindness is an English translation of the Pali word *metta*. (Pali is the language in which the Buddha's words were originally recorded in the first century BCE, 400 years after he died.) *Metta* also means "friendliness," "love," "benevolence," and "good will." In its fullest expression, *metta* is "universal, unselfish, all-embracing love." The terms *metta* and *loving-kindness* are used interchangeably in this book.

Detailed instructions for cultivating loving-kindness were first introduced by the Buddhist monk Buddhaghosa, in the 5th century CE, in the *Visuddhimagga* ("The Path of Purification"). To our knowledge, the Buddha gave only brief instructions for loving-kindness (*metta*) meditation. The way we practice metta today is essentially Buddhaghosa's elaboration of a discourse given by the Buddha to a group of monks who were afraid to live in the forest. The following lines come from that discourse:

> May all beings be happy and secure, may their hearts be wholesome!
>
> Whatever living beings there are: feeble or strong, tall, stout or medium, short, small or large, without exception; seen or unseen, those dwelling far or near, those who are born or those who are yet to be born—may all beings be happy!
>
> Let none deceive another, nor despise any person whatsoever in any place.
>
> Let one not wish any harm to another out of anger or ill-will.
>
> Just as a mother would protect her only child at the risk of her own life, even so, let one cultivate a boundless heart towards all beings.
>
> Let one's thoughts of boundless love pervade the whole world; above, below and across, without any obstruction, without any hatred, without any enmity.
>
> Whether one stands, walks, sits or lies down, as long as one is awake, one should develop mindfulness. This, they say, is the noblest living here.

The Buddha essentially prescribed loving-kindness as an antidote to fear, and he encouraged his monks to remember this discourse as a means to cultivate that quality.

It's good to keep in mind that the Buddha was a human being, not a god. When the Buddha was asked if he was a god, he simply replied that he was awake. (*Buddha* means "awake.") The Buddha was born as a prince in 563 BCE, but he left his comfortable home when he was 29 years old to discover how to overcome suffering, especially the misery associated with sickness, old age, and death. Six years later, as he was sitting under a tree in meditation, the Buddha became "enlightened"—he saw how we create suffering in our own minds and how to eliminate it. He went on to teach others for the remaining 45 years of his life.

The Buddha told his students to test everything he said on the basis of their own direct experience—"come and see." If you read the earliest Buddhist texts, you'll notice the Buddha was more of a psychologist than a religious leader. He offered a detailed map of the mind; his approach was based on objective, internal observation; and the motivation behind his words was to alleviate emotional suffering. This accounts for modern psychology's careful study of the Buddha's insights from 2,500 years ago.

In the 1960s and 1970s, as the baby boomers came of age, some intrepid Western seekers traveled to India and parts of Southeast Asia in search of new wisdom. Two such pilgrims, Sharon Salzberg and Joseph Goldstein, discovered mindfulness meditation in India. They returned home to the United States and, along with their friend Jack Kornfield, who had been a monk in Thailand, established a meditation center in rural Massachusetts. Their vision flourished. Sharon was also the first person to introduce metta meditation to a large Western audience, through her book *Lovingkindness: The Revolutionary Art of Happiness*. This classic work is an important resource for anyone interested in learning more about the subject. It takes a Western Buddhist perspective, is deeply inspirational, and contains valuable suggestions for practice.

It was Buddhaghosa who first emphasized the importance of *self*-kindness in metta practice. Buddhaghosa was careful to note that the purpose of self-kindness is to connect with our common wish to be happy, not to aggrandize the "self," which only causes more misery. When we recognize within ourselves the instinct for self-care, we're more inclined to see it in others and to work for their welfare as well.

The message of this brief history is that you should feel free to tailor the practice to fit your own needs. The Buddha didn't lay down a fixed structure or language for cultivating loving-kindness—and he wouldn't have wanted you to follow it slavishly anyway. You'll learn the basic principles of loving-kindness meditation in this chapter so that you can achieve maximum benefit from the practice.

MIXING MINDFULNESS AND METTA

Metta practice builds on the foundation of mindfulness. You'll recall that mindfulness is awareness of what's happening in the present moment. When we're upset, we're usually mind*less*—preoccupied with our personal stories ("I'm angry at Jenny because she said *this* to me and then she did *that!*")—rather than simply aware that we're in discomfort or that it *hurts* to feel that way. Mindfulness is the ability to feel our pain—if there's pain to feel—and stay out of the drama. That's step one in metta practice. When we're aware of and open to discomfort, kindness and compassion flow more easily.

It's not easy to stay open—nonresisting, nonavoiding, nonentangled—in the presence of pain. As you read in Chapters 3 and 4, mindfulness strategies can help. We can deconstruct a difficult emotion into moment-to-moment bodily experience (this twitch, that pounding heart) or we can label the emotion (anger, fear). We can also work with the direction of our awareness—inside or outside the body—to regulate the intensity of emotion. During extremely difficult periods in our lives, however, mindfulness techniques may miss the mark. When we fall to pieces, we need to be put back together again. Metta is designed to do that, especially when the practice is used in everyday life.

Loving-kindness meditation uses the power of *connection*,

whereas mindfulness meditation primarily uses *attention*. Both metta and mindfulness transform the way we relate to what's happening in our lives—they're "relational" practices—but metta focuses specifically on the *person* who's suffering. When we suffer intensely, we may need to feel held or embraced by another person. That "other person" can be a real, physical human being or, no less effectively, a compassionate part of ourselves. If we activate warmth and love within ourselves, we can often talk ourselves through difficult times. Metta meditation teaches us how to be a better friend to ourselves.

Dedicated practitioners of either mindfulness or metta eventually develop a similar state of mind—"loving awareness" or "mindful compassion." There's a Zen saying: "Kindness is the fruition of awareness, and awareness is the foundation of kindness." The film *The Lives of Others* illustrates how kindness can emerge when we pay careful attention to another person. (Spoiler alert!) In this remarkable movie, an East German secret policeman, holed up with listening devices in the attic of his prey for days on end, eventually finds himself feeling sympathetic to his enemy. That's the cost of careful attention. Have you ever wondered how therapists can listen to people's problems all day long without getting completely overwhelmed? The same principle applies: *Pay rapt attention to another person over time and the quiet energy of love and compassion will rise up.*

Loving-kindness meditation is a variation of single-focus meditation. As you'll soon see, we're using words instead of the breath as the anchor of attention. Whenever the mind wanders from the words, we note what took the mind away and return to the words. If you practice intensive metta meditation, you'll also discover a lot about your shadow side: jealousy, hatred, fear, self-judgment. You can switch seamlessly back to using your breath as an anchor for attention if the feelings become too strong.

Some people "book-end" mindfulness meditation with loving-kindness meditation. They start and end their meditation with words of kindness and compassion. That helps mindfulness practitioners go easier on themselves—to strive less and enjoy themselves more. People (like me) for whom loving-kindness is their *primary* meditation ay start meditating on the breath and the body because it stabilizes attention and calms the mind and then move on to metta practice. You'll probably discover for yourself how nicely loving-kindness and mindfulness practices complement each other.

The following exercise is the only one in this chapter. Please set aside time to do it. Read through the instructions, then put down the book, close your eyes, and give it a try. That will make the rest of the chapter much more meaningful.

TRY THIS: Loving-Kindness Meditation

Please set aside 20 minutes for the purpose of giving yourself loving attention. Sit in a comfortable position, reasonably upright and relaxed. Close your eyes and bring your attention to the heart region of your body. Now take three slow, easy breaths from the heart.

- Form an image of yourself sitting down. Note your posture on the chair as if you were seeing yourself from the outside. Feel the sensations in your body as you sit.

- Recall that every living being wants to live peacefully and happily. Connect with that deep wish: "Just as all beings wish to be happy and free from suffering, may I be happy and free from suffering." Let yourself feel the warmth of that loving intention.

- Now, keeping an image of yourself sitting in the chair and feeling good will in your heart, repeat the following phrases silently and gently:

  May I be safe.
  May I be happy.
  May I be healthy.
  May I live with ease.

- Let each phrase mean what it says. If necessary, repeat one phrase a few times for the sake of clarity. You can also repeat just one word of a phrase—"safe … safe … safe"—to experience the meaning.

- Take your time. Keep an image of yourself in your mind's eye, enjoy your loving heart, and savor the meaning of the words. When you notice that your mind has wandered, which it will do after a few seconds, repeat the phrases again. If the words become meaningless, revisualize yourself in the chair and offer yourself the phrases again. If both the image of yourself sitting and the words become vague or blurry, put your hand on your heart and recall your intention to fill yourself with loving-kindness: "Just as all beings wish to be happy and free from suffering, may I be happy and free from suffering." Then return to the phrases. Whenever you feel lost, return to the phrases.

- Let this exercise be easy. Don't try too hard. Loving-kindness is the most natural thing in the world. Distractions will always arise, and when you notice them, let them go and return to the phrases. When your attention wanders, return to giving love to yourself. Sitting with yourself is like sitting with a dear friend who's not feeling well; you may not cure your friend, but you'll have offered the kindness he or she deserves.

- Now gently open your eyes.

GOOD WILL VERSUS GOOD FEELINGS

Loving-kindness is an acquired skill. Some people seem to have a natural talent for it. The majority of us, however, are likely to find loving-kindness meditation awkward at first. Why?

The main reason for difficulty is that we have expectations about how we're supposed to feel. Fortunately, as Sharon Salzberg reminds us, "loving-kindness meditation works even if you don't feel a thing!" It works with our deepest motivation: good will. Sometimes good intentions stir up good feelings, sometimes they evoke obstacles to pleasant emotions, like self-doubt or self-judgment, and sometimes they conjure up nothing at all.

Loving-kindness practice doesn't *directly* change how we feel, but it helps us hold ourselves in a gentle way that lets emotions change by themselves. Do you remember the story of Michelle at the beginning of this book? Michelle's therapeutic challenge was to give up the wish to hide her shyness from onlookers. Loving-kindness meditation was instrumental in Michelle's recovery. By offering herself compassion first, Michelle learned to relinquish the need to control her blushing. She felt good enough about herself to risk being seen as a shy person.

Try to abandon expectations about how you should feel while doing loving-kindness meditation. If you feel discouraged by the lack of good feelings in metta meditation, bring kindness to yourself *because* you're feeling discouraged: "May I be safe, happy, healthy, and live with ease." Shift your attention away from what you want and onto how you feel, that is, "not good." With each kind word, you're planting a seed that will grow, in its own due time, into a good feeling. Intentions come first, feelings later.

Positive changes will occur when you least expect them. For example, when I first stood up to give a speech after learning metta meditation, I found myself saying, "May I and everyone here be happy and free from suffering." To my amazement, my anxiety subsided considerably. After using the metta phrases for a number of years, I've become significantly happier and less upset when things go wrong. As I said in the Introduction, self-compassion is like having a good friend around providing encouragement at just the right moments.

THE POWER OF WORDS

Words can be more powerful than actions. A broken bone can heal in a few months, but a harsh word can create a wound that doesn't heal in an entire lifetime. Most of the words we hear are actually going on *inside* us. Even if you're not generally a talkative person, your mind is constantly chattering away. If you say unkind things to yourself ("You're a worthless piece of s—t"), you'll suffer. If you say nice things ("That was *good!*"), you'll be happy. *Words shape our experience.* That's the rationale behind using words as the focus of attention in loving-kindness meditation.

Taken together, the four loving-kindness phrases comprise a kindly attitude toward a broad range of life experience. For example, if you're in danger, you'll wish for safety; if you're emotionally upset, you'll want contentment; if you're physically sick, you'll wish for health; and if you're struggling to meet everyday needs, you'll hope for fewer problems and greater ease. The metta phrases cover all this territory.

The phrases are neither exhaustive nor etched in stone. Buddhaghosa started us out almost 1,500 years ago with the following phrases: "May I be happy and free from suffering" and "May I keep myself free from enmity, affliction, and anxiety and live happily." As you understand more about the practice, you'll want to create your own phrases. Here are some examples:

May I love myself just as I am.
May I be *truly* happy.
May I find peace in this uncertain world.
May my happiness continue to grow.
May I have happiness and the causes of happiness.
May I live in peace, without too much attachment and too
      much aversion.
May I be free from sorrow.
May I be free of physical suffering.
May I care for myself with ease.
May I love and be loved.
Dear one, may you be happy and content.

The idea is to find words that evoke tender, warm feelings inside you. They can be sublime, like poetry, or mundane. It's best to keep the phrases simple and easy to repeat.

During the uprising against the repressive government of Myanmar, Buddhist monks gathered in front of the home of Aung San Suu Kyi on September 22, 2007, and chanted:

> May we be completely free from all danger.
> May we be completely free from all grief.
> May we be completely free from poverty.
> May we have peace in heart and mind.

Metta phrases incline the heart toward peace and well-being in spite of the terrible circumstances happening on the ground.

You can tailor the phrases for everyday challenges in your own life. For example, if you're caught up in shame, you can repeat, "May I accept myself just as I am." If you feel angry, try "May I be safe and free from anger." Avoid being too specific about your wishes, such as "May I get into the college of my choice!" lest your wish become a demand for a particular outcome. Loving-kindness is an inclination of heart, not an attempt to manipulate the environment with our thoughts.

In your formal meditation practice—when you sit down *specifically* to cultivate loving-kindness—try to use the *same* metta phrases again and again. Metta meditation is a focused attention practice, and your mind will be calmed by repetition alone. If you slip into a state of loving absorption, you may find a stream of new metta phrases flowing through you. That's a wonderful experience, but please use your regular phrases when you return to your ordinary frame of mind.

In addition to focusing our attention, loving-kindness meditation has a contemplative component. Contemplation meditation is a method for exploring the deeper meaning of an idea, such as reading a passage from sacred scripture and rolling it over in your mind until hidden layers are revealed. Carefully chosen metta phrases work like that; when we mull over the same words again and again, we get a direct, visceral sense of their meaning. This takes time, and we may see nothing for long periods—like waiting for tulips to emerge in the spring—but it's worth the wait.

There's a quiet joy that comes in meditation when the metta phrases and their meaning connect. You may discover that in an unexpected moment during the day, you'll find yourself thinking

Compassion Meditation and the Brain

In a study by Richard Davidson and colleagues, monks with 10,000 to 50,000 hours of practice in "non-referential compassion meditation"—"unrestricted readiness and availability to help living beings"—were compared to novices with only 1 week of training. Both groups were outfitted with a head net of 128 EEG electrodes and then began to meditate. The group of monks produced exceptionally powerful gamma waves (indicating intensely focused awareness) that were 30 times stronger than in the novice meditators, the wave patterns covered exceptionally broad areas of the monks' brains, and the wave patterns were synchronized. This unusual brain state could be quickly turned on by the experienced meditators, and it tended to linger during the rest periods rather than go into "default mode." Also, the monks with the most experience had the highest levels of gamma waves. Davidson's research demonstrates that with intense practice we can develop astonishing control over brain activity and evoke loving feelings at will, independent of an object or circumstances.

Another study in Davidson's lab was designed to detect whether brain circuits that detect emotions could be strengthened through meditation. Sixteen monks with over 10,000 hours of training in nonreferential compassion meditation were compared to 16 novices who had a 2-week training period. The meditators' brains were imaged using fMRI as they reacted to sounds (distressed woman, baby laughing, background restaurant noise). Compared to novices, the monks showed increased activity in the insula (responsible for empathy and body awareness) and the temporal parietal juncture (where emotions of others are especially perceived) in response to the sound of the distressed woman. The monks more strongly detected *all* emotional sounds—positive, negative, and neutral—suggesting that compassion meditation attunes the brain to process all sorts of emotional stimuli, not just to process suffering.

"Oh, *this* is happy!" While doing psychotherapy, perhaps while a tear is trickling down my cheek, I'll note, "Oh, this is *compassion*." There's neither pride nor embarrassment in it—just the simple experience. The loving-kindness phrases and the experience come together gradually.

What matters most is the *attitude* behind the phrases. Words may or may not reflect how we truly feel—we can fake words and try to distort reality with them. A friend of mine once remarked that loving-kindness meditation is like talking to her pet dog. You can call your dog a "miserable wretch" in a loving way and get away with it every time. You can also say "I love you" with a scowl and scare your dog under the table. Your dog isn't evaluating your choice of words; it's connecting with your intentions. I saw a bumper sticker that read "I want to be the person my dog thinks I am!" Somehow our dogs see our *deepest* intentions and forgive us our moods. In metta meditation, stick to your core motivation—to be happy and free from suffering—and don't get bogged down in the words. The more we incline the heart toward loving-kindness, the more that will be the habit our brains are exercising.

FINDING A WAY TO YOURSELF

You probably had difficulty focusing on yourself when you did loving-kindness meditation. That may be due to a naturally wandering mind, but more likely it's due to ambivalence about the process. The majority of us find it strange or difficult to give ourselves love.

Even after years of practice, I occasionally feel guilty ("This is too self-centered") when I direct metta toward myself. That comes from my childhood as well as our culture. I know that self-directed loving-kindness makes me a better person, so I remind myself, "Give yourself the attention you need so you don't need so much attention!" It was also written in the *Visuddhimagga*, "Just as I want to be happy and dread pain, as I want to live and not die, so do other beings, too." There's no need to *exclude* ourselves from loving-kindness. If you feel guilty directing loving-kindness toward yourself, ask yourself who told you that focusing on yourself was wrong or how growing up in your family taught you to care only for others.

As mentioned in the last chapter, loving ourselves is used as an *example* in religious traditions for how we should treat others. "Love your neighbor as yourself." Self-kindness is not where the process stops—it's the beginning. The joy of caring for others is ultimately deeper and longer lasting than caring for ourselves because it liberates us from a narrowly defined sense of "self." Also, as the Dalai Lama says, there are so many more opportunities to love others! But when we're in pain, as we often are, we must know how to love ourselves.

Another reason for not giving ourselves kindness is that we feel we don't deserve it. Feelings of worthlessness are lurking in almost everyone, even in *teachers* of loving-kindness.

A group of Western scientists and Buddhist teachers met with the Dalai Lama in 1990 during a conference in Dharamshala, India. Sharon Salzberg asked him, on behalf of the other meditation teachers, how they might help their students who suffered from feelings of worthlessness and shame.

The Dalai Lama didn't seem to understand the question, so he and his translator spoke back and forth on this topic. When he realized what was being asked, the Dalai Lama showed genuine surprise, and he asked the gathering whether they were certain this was *really* the case. They responded that it was a problem not only for their students but also for *themselves*. The Dalai Lama then went from person to person, inquiring, "Do you experience this? Do you?" It was hard for him to grasp that a person could actually dislike him- or herself.

I often wonder why the Dalai Lama was so surprised by this phenomenon. Research by Kristin Neff suggests that lack of self-compassion is not a unique quality of Western life. Ironically, it's precisely when we need love the most that it is hardest to give it to ourselves.

How can we use loving-kindness meditation to care for ourselves? Here are a few suggestions.

Opening to Pain

Pain helps. When we're open to pain, compassion flows like water down a mountainside. The metta phrases have an uncanny ability to soothe us when we're feeling really bad. Many people have complaints ("Too touchy-feely"; "It's just *words*") about their loving-kindness practice when they feel *good,* yet when they feel bad the phrases are deeply comforting. Metta meditation can be like a spouse who's taken for granted—until a crisis comes. Explore for yourself how differently metta meditation feels when you're happy and when you're not.

Pain is more available than you think. The body accumulates stress all day long, consciously or unconsciously. It's a myth that we know when we're under stress; usually we ignore stress as it wreaks havoc on the mind and body, shortening our lives and making our days more difficult. Here's where mindfulness comes in: Before you do metta meditation, do a quick sweep of your body and identify any places of tension. Check in with yourself emotionally too: "How am I feeling?" Acknowledge any discomfort you may be holding in your body and mind and then begin the practice.

It's a common mistake to use loving-kindness meditation to make pain go away. The first step toward relief is being aware of pain and opening to it. When you feel emotional pain in the present moment ("This *really hurts!*"), a deep, sympathetic response is likely to arise ("Oh God, may I be free from suffering!"). Alternatively, if you're battling against pain right from the start, you'll find yourself demanding, "Stop, stop, stop, *please* stop the pain!" That's perfectly understandable, but it's a lot of work and not likely to succeed.

Be patient with the practice. There's a Jewish story that illustrates how the practice works:

A disciple asks the rebbe, "Why does Torah tell us to 'place these words *upon* your hearts'? Why does it not tell us to place these holy words *in* our hearts?"

The rebbe answers, "It is because as we are, our hearts are closed, and we cannot place the holy words in our hearts. So we place them on *top* of our hearts. And there they stay until, one day, the heart breaks and the words fall in."

Pain is our ally when we have an open heart.

Finding Good Qualities

We're naturally attracted to good qualities. For example, historical figures to whom we're most drawn are the moral geniuses, not necessarily the military or political figures. Likewise, if we think of something good about ourselves, we enjoy keeping ourselves company. If we think ill of ourselves, our attention will flail around looking for distraction from these inner threats to our self-image. At the beginning of your meditation, remind yourself of one or two of your good qualities: loyalty to family, conscientiousness, kindness toward animals, perhaps a sense of humor? You'll feel more worthy of your own attention.

Loving-Kindness Builds Positive Resources

Barbara Fredrickson at the University of North Carolina and colleagues compared people who had done 7 weeks of loving-kindness meditation to a group of people on a waiting list. Metta meditation significantly increased positive emotions (such as love, joy, gratitude, hope, amusement, and awe), as well as a wide range of personal resources such as mindfulness, problem-solving ability, savoring the future, environmental mastery, self-acceptance, purpose in life, social support received, positive relations with others, and physical health. Furthermore, these increases in personal resources predicted life satisfaction and fewer symptoms of depression. During the study, practitioners of loving-kindness showed a steady gain in the number of positive emotions they experienced with each hour that they meditated—they were building a reliable skill for generating positive emotions that kept them ahead of the adaptation (hedonic treadmill) effect.

Connecting with Others

I know a woman who would give up her life for her beloved dog but who could barely feed herself. She began loving-kindness meditation for her dog, "May Ginger be happy and content," and then she tucked herself into that thought, "May Ginger *and I* be happy and content." Eventually, she could say "May *we* be happy ..." and finally "May *I* ..." Sometimes we need to *sneak up on ourselves* with kindness.

Compassion toward others can also put us in a compassionate mood toward ourselves. Think of someone you like who is suffering in a way similar to your own suffering. Then gradually step up to include yourself in the metta phrases: "May [*Sandra*] be safe and free from harm ... ," "May [*Sandra*] *and I* be safe ... ," May *we* ... ," May *I* ..." You can also start with a person you loved very much in the past, such as a child, and remember how you felt when that person was sick or in pain. Hold in your heart the natural compassion you feel and then fold yourself into the mix.

Yet another way to mobilize an affectionate attitude is to form an image of *yourself* as a young child, perhaps from an old photograph. An endearing image can inspire a loving frame of mind. You can set a childhood picture of yourself on a table and just leave it there for a few weeks, allowing yourself to contemplate it in a casual way, and then bring it into your meditation when you're ready. I have a psychotherapy client for whom an image of himself as a lonely child inspired the self-compassion he had previously been unable to find.

For some people self-kindness arises more easily if it begins abstractly: "May *all beings* be happy." Then we include ourselves: "May *I and all beings* be happy." You can also begin with greater emotional distance by using your own name: "May [*Sam*] be peaceful and happy" rather than "May *I* be peaceful and happy."

If you've had trauma in relationships and are ambivalent about people, you can meditate on a cherished object from nature like a tree or the ocean ("May *this tree* be healthy and strong"). Then gradually transition to a pet ("May *Ginger* be healthy and strong") and eventually to yourself ("May *I* ..."). The principle is this: Connect with anyone or anything that puts a smile on your face and go from there. Follow your heart and then bring yourself into the picture.

The object of your loving-kindness is less important than the *attitude* you're generating. Your brain is most likely to repeat whatever it's experiencing in each moment. If you feel stressed, you're learning stress. If you feel kindly, you're learning kindness. The rest is details.

LOVING-KINDNESS IN THREE-PART HARMONY

There are three technical components to metta practice: (1) words, (2) feelings, and (3) images. The *image* gives us a target, the *words* evoke our deepest wishes, and the *feelings* are the preverbal gut sense of what we're saying.

People find different components easier to practice than others. For example, verbal types work easily with words, sensing people go with the feelings, and visual folks easily call up images. It helps to know our own tendencies. For example, I'm a visual person and can easily hold an image in my mind. When I refresh the image of myself during meditation, the words deepen their meaning and the feelings grow stronger (including the *resistance* to kindly intentions!). The practice becomes more powerful when we emphasize the part we're good at.

Ideally, we want to get all three components of metta practice working together: words, feelings, and images. The practice can be revitalized when you *switch* between components. For example, when the words become meaningless, refresh your aim by focusing on the image. If the feeling dries up, connect with the meaning of the words—repeating them slowly and savoring what you're saying. Move back and forth from the feelings to the words to the feelings, and occasionally remind yourself of the image. Be creative in your meditation. The point is to encourage the attitude of loving-kindness to arise as much as possible.

Words

The phrases should be spoken in a tone that reflects your loving intentions—softly and gently. Give the phrases the feeling of candle-light. During informal practice in daily life, you can say the phrases out loud, chant them, or sing them along with a favorite tune, but be careful that if you are raising your voice you're doing it to *embrace* what's happening in your life, not to drive away any bad feelings.

Say the phrases slowly, letting them resonate one at a time. You can't read poetry in a rush and have it evoke something new within you. Give yourself time to contemplate what you're saying during metta practice. Don't try to accomplish anything—anything other than offering yourself kindness.

When you're deep into meditation, you might find that the complete phrases you've chosen become cumbersome. You can sim-plify them to a few key words, such as "safe, peaceful, healthy, ease," or to one word repeated over and over, like "love, love, love." Use your intuition and find words that work for you, preferably ones that are pleasant and easy to repeat.

At some point, the phrases will become empty or robotic. Any object of attention is like that: it loses its charge after sufficient rep-etition. That doesn't necessarily mean the words should be changed. Instead, stay close to the *wishing* side of the practice rather than the *feeling* side. Your core motivation is the energetic center of the prac-tice. Remind yourself *why* you're meditating: to be happy and free from suffering. See yourself as one of many beings who want a life of contentment and ease. Then fold your personal metta phrases—"May I be safe," and so on—into that wellspring of inspiration.

Another problem with the metta phrases is that they don't make sense to some people. You might ask, "How can I possibly expect happiness and ease? That's unrealistic! Aren't stress and discomfort part of everyone's life?" That's true, of course. The most difficult principle of metta practice to understand is that we're not trying to generate a particular *outcome*. A kindly attitude is its own reward. What the metta phrases really mean is the following:

- "Even though it's unrealistic to expect peace and happiness all the time, *may it be so whenever possible*."

- "I have the wish, *at this very moment,* to be healthy and free from suffering, but the future is not in my control."

The phrases should be intellectually credible—they should make sense—or the mind will quietly argue and lose concentration on the task.

Feelings

Feelings refer to the felt sense of loving-kindness. Sometimes the will to love comes with warm emotions and sometimes it doesn't. A wish is not a feeling, and our feelings are far less predictable than our wishes. We can always fall back on the *wish* for happiness, but the corresponding feelings may be few and far between.

When loving feelings are present, they can be used to strengthen our core motivation. Savor the feelings—linger over them—as long as they occur. Words are extraneous when you have a loving feeling, but as the feeling subsides, return to the words. Warm feelings are like a good meal; why turn away and have a less nutritious meal when you can enjoy a good one?

Some sensing-feeling people are better at savoring feelings than intellectual types. The more aware you are of your body, the more you'll be able to enjoy good feelings. You've already learned a number of exercises for becoming aware of the body and emotions, especially "Mindfulness of Bodily Sensations" (Chapter 2) and "Mindfulness of Emotion in the Body" (Chapter 3). Those exercises can help even the most intellectual types develop their sensing-feeling side.

Some beginning meditators can generate compassionate feel-

ings just by thinking about them, such as the experienced meditators in Richard Davidson's experiments, but that's quite rare. Usually we need to create the *conditions* for such feelings to arise. For
example, if you think of someone you love, metta will arise; if you
think of someone who's in *pain* whom you love, compassion will
arise. There's a bit of "method acting" in the feeling side of loving-
kindness practice: we enter into the present moment and allow the
phrases and images to work on us. Feelings of loving-kindness and
compassion will arise the more you practice. After many thousands
of hours, they'll follow you like a state of grace.

You can also try the following simple strategies to make yourself
receptive to loving feelings:

- Play love songs before you meditate.
- Practice in a delightful place.
- Make yourself physically comfortable.
- Relax your body.
- Put a light smile on your lips and crinkle your eyes.
- Visualize yourself in a good mood.
- Keep a pet in your lap.
- Place your hand over your heart.
- Speak the phrases from your heart.

These small modifications help to establish a warm, friendly agenda
for the rest of your meditation. Again, please don't *expect* loving feelings. We're only creating conditions for them to occur on
their own.

Images

The person on whom you focus your attention has a great impact
on whether loving-kindness will arise during your practice. At the
beginning of practice, "other people" serve to give us an easier way
to love ourselves. Meditation practitioners who are able to feel natu-

ral kindness for themselves are ahead of the game. In the next chapter, you'll explore what happens when you focus on people toward whom you have very little feeling or people who are hard to be with. Before you subject yourself to these more challenging tasks, however, you need to become skilled at awakening loving-kindness for yourself. Be patient. It's not uncommon to spend the first 2 to 3 years of metta practice just learning to love yourself.

Some suggestions were given earlier for how to connect with *other* people as a prelude to giving love to yourself. Generally speaking, start with someone who makes you smile (to cultivate friendliness) or who melts your heart (to cultivate compassion). Choose a personal relationship that's simple, pleasant, and uncomplicated. If you have a sexual relationship with the person, hidden attachment could emerge and disturb your focus. If the person has passed away, feelings of loss could creep in. Make sure the image doesn't arouse much ambivalence.

The clearer the image, the stronger the feelings that will arise. When you create an image of *yourself,* see yourself in your mind's eye in your current posture and feel your body. (You can open your eyes and look at your body, but only if that doesn't arouse self-criticism.) Make a mental note of your facial expression and remind yourself of your good qualities. Give yourself full recognition. Smile if you're inclined to. If you're focusing on another person, take some time to feel the presence of that individual with all your senses. Once you have a good, clear image, it will resonate and linger in your mind.

The most difficult person in the world to hold in loving awareness is usually oneself. We can be blindsided by unexpected, long-forgotten thoughts and feelings. A shameful way you treated your brother? An episode of infidelity in your marriage? Even when we don't like ourselves, we work with what we've got. We visualize ourselves, repeat kind wishes, savor any good feelings that the phrases evoke, refocus on our image, return to the phrases, shift to an easier person when necessary, return to ourselves, and so on. The practice requires flexibility, but we eventually learn to be affectionate with ourselves through thick and thin. By evoking good will over and over, we discover the inherent goodness behind all those disturbing thoughts, feelings, and words. This may seem like a huge achievement, but isn't that how our pets already see us? Surely we can do the same for ourselves.

BACKDRAFT

When a fire is deprived of oxygen, it will explode when fresh air is introduced through an open door. Firefighters call that "backdraft." A similar effect can occur when we practice loving-kindness. If our hearts are hot with suffering—self-hatred, self-doubt—when we begin to practice, sympathetic words can open the door of our hearts, causing an explosion of difficult feelings. Those feelings are not *created* by metta practice; we're simply recognizing and feeling them as they go out the door. It's part of the healing process.

This phenomenon is so common that my patients and others have used different metaphors to describe it:

- "Metta is like dropping cold water on a hot skillet. The water sizzles and skates around the pan. It's a good thing, but it takes time to *realize* it's a good thing."
- " 'May I be happy' is a minefield!"
- "The light of love brings up 'I'm unlovable. I'm self-indulgent.' "
- "Love is a double-edged sword; it cuts away the pain in the present, but it also slices into the pain of the past!"

Therapists are keenly aware of this process when working with people who suffer from feelings of worthlessness and shame. If a therapist says something kind or admiring, such as "You were so courageous to have challenged your father in that way," a patient struggling with low self-worth may feel mocked or patronized. That isn't due to insincerity by the therapist, but because kind words bring up negative messages from the past, like "You're nothing but a coward!" That's backdraft.

Everything we know is seen in contrast to something else. For example, we know our toe is soft because a rock is hard. For people who are full of negative thoughts about themselves, a loving remark can cause an eruption of all those contrasting ideas that, due to their intensity, feel more truthful than the kind remark. In this case, a kind comment is easily misinterpreted as an intentional insult. When it happens in meditation, we doubt our own sincerity.

We need to address the hidden feelings that erupt when we're good to ourselves in loving-kindness meditation. Do you remember the discussion of "schemas" in Chapter 4? Some of us may feel fundamentally ashamed, alone, abandoned, isolated, or deprived. These conditioned, core beliefs from childhood are guaranteed to emerge when we do loving-kindness practice. How do we work skillfully with old hurts and feelings?

The first rule is to *expect bad feelings to arise.* What comes up is *not* an obstacle to practice if you can maintain your emotional equilibrium. If sadness or grief or self-doubt arises, recognize that you're suffering in that very moment and offer yourself good will with the same phrases you've been using all along. Try not to get absorbed in the story line. Be good to yourself *because* you're feeling pain. Don't try to push away bad feelings. Focus on yourself, not on the feelings. Metta teaches you to be sympathetic toward yourself. Every moment is an opportunity to practice that, no matter what you're feeling.

The second rule is to *maintain balance.* If you find that the feelings coming up are too strong, you don't have to become more ardent in your metta practice. Don't fall into the trap of intensifying metta to fight intensely uncomfortable feelings. That's combat, not loving-kindness, and it'll only make you feel worse. Perhaps you should back off and give yourself kindness in a different, less introspective way, such as having dinner with friends or taking a trip to the beach. If you feel emotionally numb, that's a sure sign you should back off and be good to yourself in another way, perhaps by engaging in an activity described in Chapter 5.

The third rule is to *apply mindfulness.* If it makes sense to stick with your meditation, you can always switch to using your breath or another anchor (sound, touch) when the phrases generate too much feeling. Remember, however, to saturate your mindfulness practice with affection. Use the skills from Chapters 2 and 3. Try labeling the emotion ("Ah, jealousy"; "Ah, embarrassment"; "Ah, anger"). If you linger with the emotion, a tightly held emotion *behind* it may release, such as anger behind guilt or fear behind anger. When labeling is not enough, locate the sensation of the emotion in your body, perhaps in your abdomen, chest, or throat, and describe the feeling tone ("unpleasant"). Then give yourself more metta.

If a core belief, or schema, arises in meditation, you can label that too: "abandonment," "mistrust," "defectiveness," "inadequacy." Offer labels in a soft, gentle tone. Go back and forth from the primary object (the phrases) to the most compelling object of awareness (the schema). Sit in the middle of your experience, like the Zen metaphor of a lotus flower in the middle of flames. Old memories may present themselves for mindful awareness. For example, if you're a perfectionist, you might discover where you first heard that being "good enough is not good enough." If you're chronically angry, you might find yourself thinking of the person who told you that people should always be punished for their mistakes. If you're terrified of being left alone, a person who was excessively worried about you may pop into your mind. As these events occur, simply note them and return to your mental anchor.

In general, see if you can work with backdraft as you would with any distraction: note what's happening, softly and gently, and return to the phrases. Please don't make yourself suffer by trying too hard to remove your imperfections. As a wise person once said, "Attend to your sensitivity—a flower cannot be opened with a hammer."

LIKE A PRAYER

There are similarities between loving-kindness meditation and prayer. When I asked a client of mine how his metta practice was going, he replied, "This is easy. I already know how to do my prayers." Some people ask, "Can I pray to God when I wish for happiness and freedom from suffering?" The answer is "Yes, of course!" Anything that cultivates loving intentions is metta practice. But there's a catch.

I knew a woman, Paula, who suffered from hepatitis and prayed constantly to be relieved of her illness. Paula told me, "I had nothing but disappointment, so I just stopped praying." Eventually she discovered metta practice and took to it enthusiastically, mainly because she could feel the love of prayer without the trap of expecting her life to change. Metta taught her surrender—surrender of the *outcome* of her efforts. Traditional prayer can be of two types:

When Prayer Is Avoidance

Robert Zettle and colleagues from Wichita State University wanted to know whether accepting pain makes it easier to bear. Using scores on a questionnaire, participants were grouped as either experience avoiders ("Anxiety is bad") or nonavoiders ("I'm not afraid of my feelings"). Both groups were then asked to put a hand in a tray of cold water (40 degrees Fahrenheit) for up to 5 minutes. Researchers measured how long participants could keep their hands in the cold water. Afterward, participants filled out a questionnaire describing what they were thinking during the experiment.

As predicted, the nonavoiders could tolerate the cold water much longer than the avoiders, even though both groups were equally sensitive to pain. Avoidant people used unhelpful mental strategies such as catastrophizing ("It's terrible and I feel it's never going to get better") and prayer/hoping ("I pray for the pain to stop"). In short, people who can accept the experience of pain, without praying that it will go away, can endure pain for longer periods of time.

surrender ("Thy will be done") or outcome ("Please heal this disease"). Metta helped Paula discern that it's possible to hold a wish ("Dear God, *may* I ...") without a demand ("... get cured of my hepatitis!"). Surrender-type prayers don't assume that we know what's best for us or how things should be done; they're an inclination of heart rather than an effort to control or manipulate an outcome. In other words, we're holding our situation and desires a little more lightly.

Metta is secular prayer. Many people wish they had faith in a higher power, but they can't seem to get there. A client of mine said, "I'm envious of the God people!" Metta is an opportunity for theists and nontheists alike to cultivate unconditional love by staying close to their deepest wishes. In the words of the poet Galway Kinnell, "The bud stands for all things ... for everything flowers from within, of self-blessing." The bud doesn't need to appeal to something beyond itself to blossom; it's in the nature of a bud to flower. Our deepest nature will also flourish when it's fertilized with good will and loving-kindness.

OFF THE CUSHION

Loving-kindness practice takes place primarily in daily life—off the cushion or the couch. Not everyone has the temperament or the time for formal sitting meditation. If you have to make a choice between formal and informal practice, better to practice as often as possible during the 16+ hours that you're engaged in daily life. Most people don't need to do formal metta meditation to benefit greatly from the practice. Every moment of loving-kindness is brain training, no matter what posture you're in. The principles and practical suggestions given so far pertain as much to loving-kindness practice in daily life as to sitting meditation.

If you want a formal, sitting loving-kindness practice, how much time should you allocate each day? Twenty to 30 minutes of loving-kindness meditation in the morning is usually quite sufficient and sets the tone for the rest of the day. Some people find that 10 minutes is enough. In general, two short sittings are better than one long sitting (30–45 minutes) because some people find the nervous system becomes destabilized, that is, nervous or edgy, with longer sittings. Find out what works best for you.

You should remember that the brain develops a habit of doing whatever it's doing. If you stress yourself out on the cushion, the brain will develop the "sit and be stressed" habit. If you generate loving-kindness, the brain is in training to experience love. Mostly we're reinforcing the *intention* to be loving and compassionate when we practice metta meditation.

You can work with the phrases anytime, night or day. I like to repeat the metta phrases informally for a few minutes before I go to sleep and again when I wake up. In the ancient text of the *Visu-dhimagga,* it's said that metta leads to sound sleep and nice dreams and also makes the practitioner dear to others. That's not hard to understand. Our dreams are more likely to be peaceful if we go to sleep without fear or anger, and people will find it difficult (though not impossible!) to dislike us if we genuinely appreciate them.

There's no better time to discover self-compassion than when you feel really bad. The last two verses of Naomi Shihab Nye's poem *Kindness* read:

Before you know kindness as the deepest thing inside,
You must know sorrow as the other deepest thing.
You must wake up with sorrow.
You must speak to it till your voice
Catches the thread of all sorrows
And you see the size of the cloth.

Then it is only kindness that makes sense anymore,
Only kindness that ties your shoes
And sends you out into the day to mail letters and purchase bread,
Only kindness that raises its head
From the crowd of the world to say
It is I you have been looking for,
And then goes with you everywhere
Like a shadow or a friend.

A heart open to sorrow may seem like a frightening prospect, but compassion can become a constant, loving companion—a palpable presence through tough times. If you notice a hurt, perhaps an experience of failure, disappointment, or rejection, say softly to yourself, "May I be safe, may I be happy, may I be healthy, may I live with ease."

There's a close association between self-compassion and *self-forgiveness*. Forgiveness is essential in life because we make mistakes all the time. Sometimes we're put into impossible situations where people get hurt even when we do the right thing: a boss who has to fire an employee who is undermining morale, for instance, or a mother who has to stop giving money to her drug-addicted son. How do we forgive ourselves when we cause others pain, knowingly or unknowingly? The first step is to keep our hearts open to our own remorse rather than deflect it with anger or self-justification. Then we respond compassionately to ourselves, in words or deeds.

Do you remember the examples given in Chapter 1 for how problems are caused by resistance to discomfort—back pain, insomnia, relationship conflict, and speech anxiety? These common conditions are also excellent opportunities to practice loving-kindness. Metta meditation comforts the *person* who's struggling, which, in turn, changes how we relate to the specific problem. It affects the eye of the beholder. For example, if I have back pain and say to myself, "May I be safe, may I be peaceful, may I be strong, may I live with ease," the soothing I bring to myself will reduce the amount of anxiety I feel when I get a twinge of pain. We move from "anxious attention" to "loving attention"—to the path of least resistance.

If you're lying awake with insomnia, worried about the next day, try offering yourself loving-kindness *because* of your unhappiness about not sleeping. Replace the focus on sleep with attention to your sad or fearful feelings and say the metta phrases to yourself, over and over. Sleeplessness is an excellent opportunity to train your brain in something useful: self-compassion. It's meditation in the lying-down position.

When you find yourself struggling in a relationship, take a break and ask yourself what hurts so much. Is it that you don't feel seen or

Loving-Kindness Meditation Reduces Back Pain

James Carson and colleagues at the Duke University Medical School did a pilot study on loving-kindness meditation as a treatment strategy, applying it to lower back pain. He and his colleagues trained their participants in eight 90-minute group meetings weekly, and the trainees practiced metta meditation at home with audiotapes. Carson found that metta meditation reduced back pain, and the longer the participants practiced (from 10–25 minutes per day), the lower their pain level at the end of the meditation session. Longer meditations also predicted less anger the following day. One participant in the study who tended to lose her temper with her debilitated, elderly mother reported, "When I enter her room now, I can feel myself soften." A businessman remarked, "I never knew it was possible to have such space in my heart for others."

heard, or you feel disrespected? Know that you deserve to be happy and free from suffering. Can you name the feeling you're having? Give yourself the love and connection you need, right there in that moment, perhaps by using the metta phrases. Then, when you feel a little better, turn to your partner and talk.

If you suffer from public-speaking anxiety, offer loving-kindness to both yourself and your audience when you go up on stage, or beforehand when you *think* about going on stage. ("May we *all* be happy and free from suffering.") Your audience might just respond to your compassionate frame of mind with compassion for your speech making! If you let yourself be just as anxious as you are, you might forget you were ever anxious. As Thomas Merton wrote, interpreting Chuang Tzu, the Taoist sage:

So, when the shoe fits
The foot is forgotten,
When the belt fits
The belly is forgotten,
When the heart is right
"For" and "against" are forgotten.

WHAT METTA IS NOT

Now that you have a preliminary understanding of loving-kindness practice, let's review what it's *not* in order to keep the practice from becoming unnecessarily complicated. It's not:

- *Selfish.* The first step toward loving others is to love ourselves. The fault we find with ourselves will also be found in others. Metta teaches us to be kind to ourselves no matter what happens, even as we shape our behavior for the better.

- *Complacent.* Metta is a force of will—good will—that can override the instinctive tendencies of fear and anger. Metta frees us from old habits. It allows us to learn from pain and respond skillfully.

- *Positive affirmation.* Affirmations are an effort to encourage ourselves by saying things we may not believe, like "I'm getting stronger every day!" Metta isn't fooling ourselves that our situation is better than it is. The phrases must be intellectually credible to work smoothly.

- *Just a mantra.* Although the metta phrases are repeated like a mantra, there's more to it than that. In addition to using the power of *attention,* metta works with *connection, intention,* and *emotion* (discussed further in the next chapter). We're doing whatever it takes to cultivate a loving attitude.

- *Sugarcoating.* We're not trying to make the reality of our lives less harsh by learning to think or speak in a sweet way. Rather, we want to open to the depth of human experience, including the tragedy of it, more fully. This is possible only if we have a compassionate response to pain.

- *A pity party.* Opening to pain is not self-indulgent. We're not wallowing in discomfort, complaining, or whining excessively. On the contrary, opening to pain through compassion allows us to unhook from the familiar story lines of our lives.

- *Good feelings.* Metta is primarily cultivation of good will rather than good feelings. Feelings come and go, but the ground of our being is the universal wish to be happy and free from suffering. That's where we put our trust.

- *Exhausting.* Exhaustion is the result of attachment—wanting things to be one way and not the other. Loving-kindness and compassion stay away from the business of controlling reality so it's more of a relief than a struggle.

- *Demanding.* Metta is always on the *wishing* side of the equation rather than the outcome side. Positive outcomes will certainly come with time, but we're primarily learning to cultivate a kind attitude no matter what happens to us or to others. Sticking with the wish and remaining unattached to the outcome is unconditional love.

I hope you'll discover how to make loving-kindness practice a natural part of your day. The practice is deceptively simple, but it's important to bring curiosity and flexibility to the matter. The guidelines given here are only a starting point. Follow your heart and, as Sharon Salzberg says, "See what happens."

Next we'll turn our attention to others, especially those nettlesome characters who take up residence in our minds when we least expect or want them to.

7

caring for others

High levels of compassion are nothing but an advanced state of self-interest.

—Tenzin Gyatso, *the 14th Dalai Lama*

This chapter will take what you've learned about caring for yourself and bring it to other relationships—the source of so much pain and joy in life. As you'll see, self-compassion is an essential, often unrecognized, ingredient in maintaining healthy relationships.

Some of you are already practicing loving-kindness meditation with other people, such as the beloved person who naturally makes you smile. But what about the difficult people in your life? Those folks can be a huge challenge to mindfulness and self-compassion. They also present you with an opportunity to deepen the practice. In this chapter, you'll learn a systematic method for transforming your relationships with others, based on respect and care for yourself.

Most of us find that giving kindness to others is easier and more palatable than loving ourselves. Some readers may still need special permission to focus on their own emotional needs. If you're among them, this chapter on caring for others could feel like a sellout. Don't worry; you'll learn here how to keep yourself in the picture even in the midst of intense and conflicting demands by other people.

"But can't I just *avoid* the people who bother me?" Although it's often a good idea to steer clear of problematic people, it's not an effective strategy overall. Unless we're hermits, we'll have to deal with difficult people on the street, in a taxicab, at the grocery store, at work, at family reunions—just about everywhere. In the immortal words of British author Douglas Adams, "People are a problem."

And unfortunately people live in our heads as well. Even if you stand alone on a mountaintop, your mind will be chattering with other people. What's the conversation you're having with your mother-in-law, your stepfather, your sister, or your friend? How does it feel? We're the first to feel the pain of our own negative emotions, as expressed in the Chinese proverb "Hatred corrodes the vessel in which it's stored."

Changing our relationships to the people in our heads is the first step toward working with them in real time. After practicing loving-kindness meditation for 3 days on Rajiv, a surly middle-aged clerk at my neighborhood convenience store, I went there late at night to buy some milk. Seeing him as I walked through the door, I broke into a spontaneous smile. My previous habit was to pay my bill and leave as soon as possible, but this time I hung around and we chatted a bit. Only when I got home did I realize what had happened. By meditating on the struggle of this man living far from his native country, working late into the night selling lottery tickets to unhappy people, my aversion had quietly turned to curiosity and caring. Rajiv was none the wiser for my efforts. Transforming relationships with others starts with us; it's an inside job.

Experiences like this gave me the confidence to tackle more difficult characters in my life. Some people make me feel guilty, some make me angry, others trigger regret or longing. One by one they've yielded to the force of inner kindness: "Just as I want to be happy and free from suffering, so does _____ want to be happy and free from suffering." Negative feelings toward others tend to separate us from ourselves and from others—they trigger aversion. Practicing loving-kindness for others has gradually made me feel less alone and more connected to life in general.

In the words of the Buddha:

> Looking after oneself, one looks after others.
> Looking after others, one looks after oneself.

What we think, feel, and do toward others shapes how we feel inside.

A heads-up: Please don't try to get through this chapter in one sitting. The first section explains why loving-kindness toward others is important and how to do it; the second section goes into concerns that might show up as you do the practice; and the third section describes how to bring the practice into your daily life. I recommend that you be a "student-practitioner": Read a section, try the practice, and then alternate your practice with some more reading for the rest of the week. Go slowly—mindful self-compassion builds gradually. A full course of loving-kindness meditation, such as described in this chapter and the preceding one, is best taught in a relaxed retreat setting over a 4- to 6-week period.

THE WAY OF CONNECTION

Loving-kindness meditation has four healing elements: *intention, attention, emotion,* and *connection.* Boosting our core intention ("May all beings be happy") brings energy and meaning into our lives, focused attention calms the mind ("Return to the phrases again and again"), positive emotions (compassion, love, tenderness) make us happy, and connection makes us feel more peaceful and secure (less alone, less afraid, with a sense of common humanity). You were introduced to self-to-self connection in the previous chapters; now you'll learn how to practice self-to-other connection. The connection element of loving-kindness practice becomes particularly apparent when we direct our attention toward others. It soothes the pain of disconnection.

Most people don't appreciate the role of connection in their lives. It's invisible. As my friend and colleague Jan Surrey explains, connection has an ebb and flow—we continually connect and dis-connect—but we're usually too preoccupied by our families, jobs, and other responsibilities to notice. That doesn't mean we don't feel it. *Disconnection hurts.* A disconnection can be subtle, such as when your partner falls asleep before you do, or it can have the devastating impact of marital infidelity or abuse.

Usually disconnection occurs under the radar. It may show up as irritability, self-doubt, worry, or sadness. When you feel lonely and disconnected, a colleague at work can become irresistibly sexy, especially while you are both working late at the office, or you may consume too much food, spend a lot of time shopping, surf the Web looking for love, or drink too much. That's when you should fol-low Jimmy Carter's advice and look for "the things you cannot see." Is disconnection what's really making you anxious? Angry? Sad? Sexually aroused? Do you feel like your old self when your spouse returns from a business trip? Or does your mood get *worse* because you feel more disconnected in the company of your partner?

Disconnections are inevitable, even in the best relationships. We're *all* incompatible to some extent. That's easy to imagine because we have different DNA, our childhood experiences are dif-ferent, and we live (or lived) in diverse economic, racial, ethnic, and gender groups. Our dreams continually collide with those of others. Therefore, every relationship includes the pain of disconnection.

Yet at the deepest level, way beyond ordinary awareness, we're all woven into the same cloth. Thich Nhat Hanh, a prominent med-itation teacher, illustrates this point in a lovely way:

> If you are a poet, you will see clearly that there is a cloud floating in this sheet of paper. Without a cloud there will be no water; without water the trees cannot grow; and without trees, you cannot make paper. So the cloud is in here. The existence of this page is dependent on the existence of a cloud. Paper and cloud are so close. Let us think of other things, like sunshine. Sunshine is very important because the forest cannot grow without sunshine, and we as humans cannot

Disconnection and Culture

About 60 million Americans—20% of the population—suffer from loneliness. Culture plays a role in how connected we feel. Ami Rokach of York University in Canada did a survey and found that both men and women in North America were lonelier than their counterparts in Spain on the dimensions of emotional distress, social inadequacy and alienation, growth and discovery, interpersonal isolation, and self-alienation.

Americans may also be losing confidence in the trustworthiness of others, another sign of loneliness. Wendy Rahn and John Transue found that social trust among high school seniors declined between 1976–1995. For example, 32% of students in 1976 felt that people in general could be trusted, whereas that percentage dropped to 17% in 1995. People were also viewed by these young adults as less helpful and less fair over the intervening years. Isolation and lack of trust reflect erosion of social connections.

Alan Hedge at Cornell University speculates that job insecurity and the relative lack of social programs like health care, pensions, and education in the United States may contribute to making Americans a "nomadic society on this treadmill"—needing to emphasize work and material security over personal connections.

grow without sunshine. So the logger needs sunshine in order to cut the tree, and the tree needs sunshine in this sheet of paper. And if you look more deeply ... you see not only the cloud and the sunshine in it, but that everything is here, the wheat that became the bread for the logger to eat, the logger's father—everything is in this sheet of paper. ... The presence of this tiny sheet of paper proves the presence of the whole cosmos.

The astronomer Carl Sagan echoes this vision: "If you wish to make an apple pie from scratch, you must first invent the universe."

Feeling separate from others is at odds with our deepest sense of self. That's why it hurts. It would be blissful indeed to have an

Hard-Wired for Empathy

The building blocks for empathizing with other people are the "mirror neurons," located primarily in the insula (empathy and internal perception) and the premotor strip (planning movement) of the brain. Mirror neurons mimic motor neurons—the ones that control our muscles. The way empathy seems to occur is that when you see another person's face, the mirror neurons will mimic what you see so you can feel what the other person is feeling. For example, if you see a person smile, the mirror neurons will make your face muscles smile and then you will feel yourself smiling and recognize what the other person is feeling. People with less active mirror neurons, such as those with autism, have difficulty understanding what's happening between characters in a movie or "reading between the lines" when engaged with other people. The implications of this research has been nicely described in Daniel Goleman's *Social Intelligence: The New Science of Human Relationships*, which builds on his earlier work on emotional intelligence.

Our mirror neurons start firing as soon as we focus on another person. Happy or unhappy? Friend or foe? We can often detect tiny changes in facial expression or verbal tone that reveal how another person is feeling, even though we're not fully aware of it. If I'm mad at my wife but plan to speak rationally and reasonably with her, my true feelings may still leak out. I might glance for a split-second too long or frown when I should have smiled. Then she says, slightly annoyed, "Why are you so testy?" and I think, "*Me?* Why are *you* so testy?" Our mirror neurons would have been communicating with each other all along despite my best efforts to hide how I feel. That's probably why it's so hard to discuss problems in a relationship; if you raise a topic when you feel unhappy, or start feeling bad after the topic is raised, your partner instantly feels as bad as you do.

The insula is full of mirror neurons that help us know what other people are feeling and intending to do. Research (mentioned earlier) has shown that both mindfulness and metta meditation activate the insula. Daniel Siegel puts these findings together in his thought-provoking book *The Mindful Brain*, suggesting that when we meditate in private, we're actually improving our capacity for connected relationships in the real world.

unbroken sense of connection with one's children, one's partner, all of one's friends, and with all people of different races, cultures, ages, and sex, and with all living creatures, no matter how much their survival needs compete with ours.

In the words of Albert Einstein:

> A human being is a part of the whole called by us "universe," a part limited in time and space. He experiences himself, his thoughts and feeling as something separated from the rest—a kind of optical delusion of his consciousness. This delusion is a kind of prison for us, restricting us to our personal desires and to affection for a few persons nearest to us. Our task must be to free ourselves from this prison by widening our circle of compassion to embrace all living creatures and the whole of nature in its beauty.

Is that possible? Well, sort of. We can feel connected even in the midst of disconnection by *not abandoning ourselves* in moments of pain. For example, it takes a lot of self-awareness and self-confidence to admit to oneself, after being snubbed by a boyfriend, "He's just not that into you!" By not dodging what we're feeling inside, we can continue to look others straight in the eye. The story of Michael and Suzanne in Chapter 1 also illustrates how bearing witness to one's own relational suffering keeps us engaged.

METTA FOR OTHERS

Once you decide it's worth developing loving-kindness toward others, basic training is necessary to deal with difficult people: income tax auditors, ex-spouses, telephone solicitors, and so on. Formal loving-kindness meditation is training for the real world. It transforms us by simultaneously exposing our emotional baggage as we reinforce the habits of loving-kindness and compassion. For example, a close friend may make you secretly green with envy if he gets a huge raise at work, or you might be angry at your sister for becoming pregnant before you did. When you start to meditate—cultivate the wish that your friend or sister be happy and free from suffering—you'll immediately come face-to-face with these contrary emotions. It helps to make peace with them before you actually *meet* face-to-face, so no one feels hurt or rejected.

There are traditionally six categories of people with whom we train ourselves in the art of loving-kindness. The trick is to start with an easy target, reinforce the loving-kindness habit, and work up from there.

1. *Self*—Your personal identity, usually located within the skin.

2. *Benefactor*—Someone who makes you consistently smile, such as a mentor, a child, a spiritual guide, a pet, or a piece of nature.

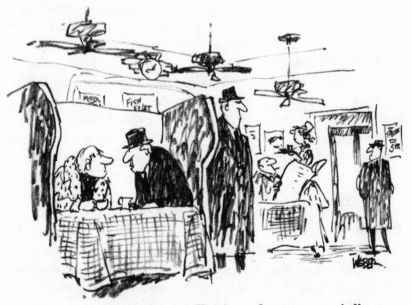

"I've got a little job for you, Kretchmer. I want you to infiltrate the I.R.S. and sow the seeds of compassion."

3. *Friend*—A supportive person toward whom you feel trust and gratitude and have mostly positive feelings.

4. *Neutral*—Any living being whom you don't know and therefore neither like nor dislike.

5. *Difficult*—Someone who has caused you pain, or toward whom you have negative feelings.

6. *Groups*—Any group of living beings, for example, everybody listed above, everyone in your home, workplace, or city.

In the preceding chapter, you were introduced to loving-kindness meditation toward the self. Some of you have also been practicing with the "benefactor" as a route to yourself. For those of you who have not yet tried the "benefactor," we'll begin there and move forward in sequence to the other categories. Once you've mastered the "difficult person," you're ready to expand loving-kindness to everyone.

To get a sense of the practice as a whole and to keep it interesting, I suggest that you try one category each day in a 20-minute meditation. Then go back and work with each category for an entire week. Please consider this chapter an *introduction* to loving-kindness meditation. If you wish to practice more intensively—longer than 20 minutes a day—please consider finding a qualified teacher. A teacher is someone who has gone down the road before you, knows the obstacles, and can guide you through them. Retreat centers and other opportunities for additional training are listed in Appendix C.

Benefactor

This category starts the process of paying careful attention to another person. The benefactor is someone who puts a smile on your face and warmth in your heart. It could be a beloved teacher, a spiritual guide, a child, a pet, or something you love in nature. Pick a relationship that's least likely to disappoint you later on—someone or something that makes you *consistently* happy.

TRY THIS: *The Benefactor*

This meditation will take 20 minutes. Begin metta meditation as described in Chapter 6: bring your attention to your heart region, take a few breaths, form an image of yourself in the sitting position, and recall that *all* beings wish to be happy and free from suffering. Then start repeating the phrases for yourself for 5 minutes or begin straightaway with your benefactor.

- Bring the benefactor's image clearly to mind and let yourself feel what it's like to be in that person's presence. Allow yourself to enjoy the good company. Also, recognize how vulnerable your benefactor is—just like you, subject to sickness, old age, and death.

- Say to yourself, "Just as I wish to be happy and free from suffering, may you be happy and free from suffering."

- Repeat softly and gently, feeling the importance of your words:

  May you be safe.
  May you be happy.
  May you be healthy.
  May you live with ease.

- When you notice that your mind has wandered, return to the words and the image of your benefactor. Linger with any warm feelings that may arise. Go slow. If you want to return to yourself, feel free to do that at any time and then switch back to your benefactor when you're ready.

- After 20 minutes, and before you end the meditation, say:

  May I and all beings be safe.
  May I and all beings be happy.
  May I and all beings be healthy.
  May I and all beings live with ease.

- Gently open your eyes.

Compared to practicing metta meditation toward yourself, focusing on the benefactor is generally pleasant and easy. But if it's the first time you've focused on the benefactor, you could have mixed feelings about the exercise. For example, you may not feel entitled to that level of intimacy with this special person, or it may feel like you're peeking in someone's window. Your reticence will probably subside over the coming week, but feel free to switch back to yourself when you need to, or return to the practice of mindfulness meditation—noticing what you're feeling while you're feeling it, with acceptance.

Friend

After working with your benefactor for a week or so, you're probably ready to move on to the "friend" category. Friends have built trust for one another over the years and feel gratitude for the relationship. The relationship is close and predominantly positive. Select a few friends and briefly audition each one with the practice instructions given above for the benefactor, using the image of your friend. You don't need to find the *perfect* friend—that doesn't exist. Most will do just fine, wrinkles and all. When you've settled on someone, work with the person for the whole week. Start each meditation with yourself as the object of meditation, go to the benefactor for a minute (or switch around the benefactor and yourself), and then move on to your friend.

Difficult feelings will invariably emerge. If you dearly love your friend, the phrase "May you be safe" could trigger anxiety that he or she may *not* be safe. Anger may arise, perhaps a memory that your friend didn't visit you in the hospital after your operation. Or you might feel envious that your friend has more money than you or has a happier marriage. When negative emotions hijack your attention, gently return to the metta phrases. If they dominate your attention, drop back to metta for yourself or your benefactor. Any unpleasant emotion—fear, anger, jealousy, shame, or remorse—is a valid reason for loving yourself.

A confusing feeling that everyone experiences from time to

time with friends is *schadenfreude*. That's the German word for feeling happy when others are going through difficulties. Ironically, a burst of joy when you hear of a close friend's good fortune may be *less* common than the schadenfreude reaction. Instead of feeling ashamed when you feel this way, just continue to cultivate loving-kindness and compassion.

Feeling disconnected is the root of schadenfreude, but our metta practice helps us feel connected. When you know you're sharing in your friend's life journey—not feeling left out—schadenfreude will yield to happiness. Say "May *she and I* be …" You'll be even happier if you can *support* your friend's achievements: "May your good fortune grow and grow." Keep saying the phrases and see what happens.

Metta Changes the Brain, Making Us More Compassionate

In a pilot study, Richard Davidson and his colleagues at the University of Wisconsin trained a group of people via the Internet to practice metta meditation for 30 minutes a day for 2 weeks. A comparison group of people learned to "cognitively reappraise" situations in their lives. After 2 weeks, only the metta group showed significant improvement on the Self-Compassion Scale (see Chapter 4). Then Davidson exposed the participants to images of human suffering, such as a child with an eye tumor, as he scanned their brains with fMRI. The metta group had increased activity in the insula (which shows empathy). The more active the insula was while the participants looked at the distressing photographs, the higher their scores on self-report scales of well-being and self-compassion. Davidson then gave the subjects the chance to donate their $165 honorarium to a cause of their choosing. Activation in the insula predicted how much money the subjects donated! This study demonstrates that only 2 weeks of loving-kindness meditation can change brain activity, make people feel more compassionate toward themselves and others, and even elicit generosity.

Loving-Kindness toward Strangers

Researchers at Stanford University found that only 7 minutes of loving-kindness meditation increased positive feelings and a sense of connection with neutral individuals. Ninety-three participants were randomly assigned to an experimental loving-kindness meditation condition or a comparable imagery condition. The loving-kindness instruction was to imagine two loved ones standing to either side of oneself sending their love. Then the participant opened his or her eyes and repeated phrases to a neutral photograph, wishing health, happiness, and well-being. The comparison condition imagined acquaintances standing in the same positions while focusing on their appearance, and later they focused on the appearance of the neutral person in the photograph. The loving-kindness group showed a significant shift toward positive responding—feeling more connected, similar, and positive toward the neutral person in the photograph.

Neutral Person

This is a very interesting category despite its dull name. It's an opportunity to develop loving-kindness toward any of the 6.7 billion people (and counting) you may encounter in your lifetime. The neutral person is someone you don't know yet, which means you have relatively little liking or disliking beyond the usual stereotypes and prejudices.

It's fun to select someone you'll probably see again so that you can gauge the effect of your meditation. That's what I did in the example of Rajiv given earlier. As the weeks progress, also remember to include animals and plants in your circle of kindness. I practiced metta for fruit flies in my kitchen while I was writing this book and had an unexpected flash of compassion when one flew in my nose. Neutral doesn't stay neutral very long when we make it the object of loving-kindness.

Your main challenge with the neutral person will be to maintain the energy of loving-kindness. You can drop back to your benefactor or yourself whenever the practice needs refreshing. Don't let the practice become dull or you'll be training your brain in the fine art of dullness. Visualize the neutral person as best you can, experience the presence of that person, repeat the words slowly and gently, sense the importance of the words, and remind yourself that the neutral person is a vulnerable being just like you, subject to pain and death.

Difficult Person

Whereas the neutral person is an exercise in *breadth,* the difficult person is an exercise in *depth.* We need to drop to a deeper place within ourselves to evoke and sustain loving-kindness toward those who've hurt us. Difficult people are therefore our "best friends" on the path of loving-kindness.

To begin with, choose a person who is *mildly* difficult, not a person who has hurt you badly or who is causing massive hardship on the world stage. Let it be someone you feel comfortable enough visualizing in meditation.

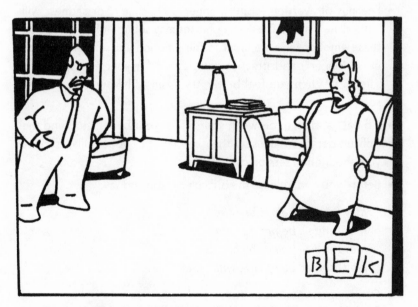

"Yeah, well, the Dalai Lama never had to deal with your whining."

TRY THIS: The Difficult Person

This meditation will also take 20 minutes. Prepare for meditation in the manner described earlier and then begin repeating the metta phrases to yourself and your benefactor (in either order) for about 5 minutes.

- Bring an image of your "difficult person" to mind. Remind yourself that the difficult person is struggling to find his or her way through life and, in so doing, is causing you pain. Say to yourself, "Just as I wish to be peaceful and free from suffering, may you too find inner peace."

- Repeat the phrases softly, keeping the image of the difficult person in your mind while sensing the value of your words:

  May you be safe.
  May you be happy.
  May you be healthy.
  May you live with ease.

- Feelings of aversion, disgust, anger, guilt, shame, or sadness will immediately arise. The metta phrases may sound hollow alongside these emotions. Give a label to the emotion you're feeling ("sadness," "anger") and practice compassion for yourself ("May I be safe …"). When you feel better, try again with your difficult person.

- Go back and forth between yourself (or your benefactor) and the difficult person. Make sure the experience of good will describes your meditation session overall.

- Before you end, release the difficult person and say:

  May I and all beings be safe.
  May I and all beings be happy.
  May I and all beings be healthy.
  May I and all beings live with ease.

- Gently open your eyes.

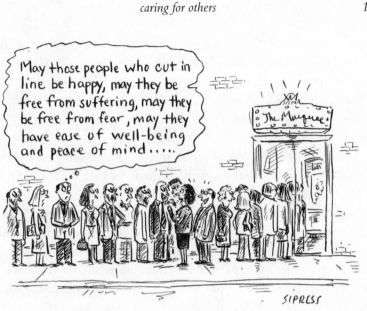

Give yourself credit for taking on this challenge. It reflects your commitment to bringing loving-kindness to all aspects of your life.

You may have the following thoughts as you work with difficult people in your life:

• *"I don't want my difficult person to be happy. Then he (or she) won't change!"* When we offer a difficult person loving-kindness, we're not accepting bad behavior or hoping the person will escape the consequences of his or her actions. Rather, we're wishing for the person to become a happy, peaceful human being. It may help to make the phrases more credible to your ear, such as, "May [Michael] heal his inner wounds and find the way to happiness." Your difficult person might change for the better when you have a warmer attitude, but try not to make your practice contingent upon his or her behavior.

• *"I don't even want to* think *about my difficult person!"* Most people instinctively wish that their difficult person would just disappear or die. There's a Tibetan saying: "Don't bother wishing your enemies will die; they'll do that anyway!" If you're having strong feelings of aversion and they don't subside, switch to a *less* difficult person. Also, don't feel obligated to feel the *presence* of the difficult person while doing metta meditation, as you would the benefactor, if it's too uncomfortable. Work with the phrases so you feel at ease and loving-kindness prevails. You might prefer the emotional distance of using a person's proper name—"May [John Doe] find inner peace …"—rather than an informal pronoun, "May *you* be …" Finally, you can always take refuge in the company of your benefactor (or your own company) whenever you wish.

• *"I spend too much time giving loving-kindness and compassion to myself!"* That's impossible. Don't worry if your meditation on the difficult person is 95% self-metta. Working with disturbing emotions ("backdraft") can comprise the majority of metta practice with difficult people. The more pain you feel, the more self-care you'll need. Sometimes it helps to put your hand on your heart and slowly breathe through your heart to get the feeling of self-compassion.

• *"Can't I start by tackling the toughest character in my life first?"* It's usually best to take a middle path—someone not too hard and not too easy. With steady practice, even the most difficult people will lose their grip on you. Use your intuition to decide whether the most difficult person will derail you from the task of generating loving-kindness.

• *"I just want to forgive and forget."* Don't rush forgiveness. Forgiveness toward others can come only after you've opened to your own pain and accepted it fully. When you feel ready, try repeating forgiveness phrases such as:

I've suffered terrible loss, fear, and self-doubt. I've been lonely and confused. I forgive myself for what I've done, knowingly or unknowingly, to harm you.

Then shift to the difficult person:

I know that you too have suffered. You've also had times of loneliness, heartache, despair, and confusion. I forgive you for what you've done, knowingly or unknowingly, to hurt me.

Repeat the forgiveness phrases as you would the metta phrases, always returning to self-metta when needed. Forgiveness requires that we deal directly with emotional pain, not bypass it.

I know a woman, Miranda, who was sexually abused in childhood by her uncle. After he committed suicide in his mid-70s, Miranda was told by her meditation teacher to meditate on the good things that her deceased uncle had brought into her life, such as creativity and reckless abandon. To her amazement, it helped Miranda heal the bitterness and despair she felt toward her uncle. This approach is generally *not* recommended until much has been done to validate one's own suffering, as Miranda had done. In her case, the teacher was also very loving and aware of how Miranda had suffered, which provided a safety net from which she could forgive her uncle. Even so, Miranda had to intermittently stop her metta practice, or focus only on herself, when she got lost in her traumatic memories.

- *"We're both good people, but the* relationship *is a pain."* You can care for the relationship as an entity, not just the participants as separate individuals. A relationship is a "we." Loving-kindness toward a relationship assumes you have made peace with yourself and the other person already. It's a slightly advanced practice. When you're ready, you can practice by saying "May *we* be safe, May *we* be happy, May *we* be healthy, May *we* live with ease."
- *"What if our culture is the 'difficult person'?"* Emotional pain is often embedded in social problems, such as racism, sexism, homophobia, and other forms of prejudice. These can also be addressed in your metta phrases: "May you and I be free from the pain of prejudice." Since prejudice is the result of ignorance, you can also try the words "May we all be free from the pain of ignorance." Both sides of the bigotry equation avoid one another to feel safe or more comfortable. The inner work of loving-kindness and compassion practice can start the process of humanizing and reconnecting with one another.
- *"Can I skip a category or stay longer with a particular person?"* The

categories are guidelines, not rules. Use your intuition and common sense, keeping the energy of loving-kindness as alive as possible. Toward that end, you can practice any way you see fit.

Groups

The final category is good will toward numerous individuals at the same time. We already practice this way at the end of each meditation session to expand the circle of loving-kindness: "May I and all beings be happy and free from suffering."

Once you've worked with all the different categories, try gathering everyone together in your mind and offering them loving-kindness at the same time. Or, as if you were hosting a dinner party, you can silently say to each person in sequence, "May you be safe ... may *you* be safe ... and may *you* be safe ..." and so on. Don't forget yourself. The guests at my party might include the Dalai Lama, a childhood friend, the clerk at the convenience store, and a politician who particularly offends me. It's fun to imagine this unlikely gathering in one place. Your "group" will be easier to visualize the longer you work with each individual in meditation.

Allow yourself to appreciate the common humanity of all the people you've gathered together. Everyone is breathing; all experience similar human emotions; everyone suffers from time to time; they all wish to be happy; and no one will live forever. Wish everyone well: "May you be safe, peaceful, healthy, and live with ease."

Other groupings can be made of the people in your home, town, country, or the entire world. You can focus on all the living beings in each of the four directions; all beings above (birds) and below (bugs and worms); all living things seen and unseen; all men and all women; all tall and short people; slim and fat; old and young. You can make up your own pairs of opposites. The "group" idea is to recognize the equality of all beings and not to exclude anyone, especially those you might tend to overlook. It's an especially expansive and joyful practice once you get the knack of it.

LOVING OTHERS WITHOUT LOSING YOURSELF

Each individual needs to find a healthy balance between self-care and caring for others, between having an authentic, personal voice and staying connected, and between the need for solitude and the need for relationship. For example, after a day of caring for her two young children, the *last* thing a woman may want is sex with her partner. What she may really need is a quiet, solitary walk or to *receive* some thoughtful attention. How do we love others without losing ourselves?

People differ in how much they enjoy connecting with others. Women seem to have a greater appetite for connection than men do. They also seem to like metta meditation more. I've even heard some men, but rarely a woman, say, "I hate metta!" Whether you're male or female, try to know, accept, and trust your own personal tolerance for connection.

During my clinical psychology internship back in 1981, I mentioned to my supervisor that I had a nightmare of people climbing through the windows of my apartment. She replied, "I think you need a vacation!" The same dream has recurred over the last 28 years whenever I need more privacy. Curiously, it happened again on a 7-day metta meditation retreat in which the participants never spoke to one another, nor did they even make eye contact. This taught me how "connected" loving-kindness meditation really is —how the head can get filled with relationships like in daily life. Taking the hint from my dream, I sought the solitude of self-metta and mindfulness practice until I was ready to "reconnect."

When Me? When Others?

When you're in pain, give yourself compassion first. Heal the healer. Sometimes a micro-moment of self-compassion is all it takes.

Take the typical morning in an American family. Under time pressure to prepare the kids for school, Mom or Dad may not recognize his or her rising stress level and inadvertently blurt out something like "Why are you *always* so unhelpful, Sean?" When that happens, try to soften into the catastrophe of the moment. Think for a second, "Ah, stress" and then say, "May I be peaceful. May I be at ease. May we *all* be peaceful and at ease." Even *before* you get up in the morning, start repeating the phrases. Then keep yourself in the picture by using the phrases whenever you need them.

As mentioned earlier, what distinguishes compassion from loving-kindness is the presence of pain. Compassion is a kindly response to *pain*. You can practice compassion for your own pain, for the pain of others, or for the pain *you* feel when *others* are in pain. Just think how you feel when images of burning homes, disemboweled bodies, and malnourished children are beamed into your home on the television. The evening news is a great opportunity to practice metta. Stay mindful of your inner state ("This is painful to watch!") and offer compassion to yourself and those on the screen ("May *I* be safe. May *you* be safe. May *we all* be safe and live in peace"). Try the same practice when you visit a friend at the hospital. Transforming your "worried attention" into "compassionate attention" through metta practice always comes as a welcome relief.

The most natural time to practice *loving-kindness* toward others is when you're genuinely happy—when you have loving energy to spare. It's easy to wish happiness for others when we're happy. You'll feel even *greater* happiness when you do so, perhaps because you're temporarily escaping the prison of your individuality by thinking of others. But timing is everything; when emotional resources are low, it's still best to focus on yourself.

Feeling shy or anxious in social situations, which everyone does from time to time, is another excellent opportunity to practice loving-kindness toward others. Why *others* at this time? A shy person is likely to be talking with an interesting person at a party and at the same time worrying whether he or she looks nervous. People feel abandoned when their conversation partners are self-absorbed. Ironically, it's the *disconnection* from a listener, rather than anxiety itself, that makes shyness such a problem. To stay in connection despite feeling anxious, try loving-kindness. When you notice yourself absorbed in your own anxiety, look the other person in the eye and think, "May *you and I* be happy." Practicing like this can help you feel less afraid on a job interview or a first date too.

Metta for others can also be used to heal disconnection in *old* relationships. Are you tired of another person "taking space in your head without paying rent" (an Alcoholics Anonymous expression)? Healing old wounds requires that we offer compassion to *both* sides of the relationship.

Helen had been divorced for 25 years and had never remarried. Her ex-husband, John, had an affair that broke up the marriage and he subsequently married that person. As Helen approached her 75th birthday, she decided she couldn't carry her angry thoughts around any longer—she didn't want to share her deathbed with bitterness. With this determination, Helen set about loosening the grip of her anger.

Helen decided to revisit in her mind how traumatic the affair and divorce had been for her and her family so many years earlier. As she did this, she comforted herself with metta phrases: "May I be safe and may I find peace." She practiced like this, over and over, for 9 months. Helen also forgave herself for her own part in the divorce: "May I forgive myself for everything I did to undermine our marriage." She addressed John in a similar way: "May I forgive you for what you did, mostly out of confusion from a life riddled with loss and abandonment, that hurt me and our family." As Helen gradually released her bitterness, her relationship with her ex-husband improved. When John died 6 years later, Helen attended the funeral and met his second wife, with very little anger remaining.

It takes courage to heal an old, troubled relationship, but, like Helen, we first need to see how *not* addressing it can be more damaging. Loving our enemies is not a moral prescription—it's just the best thing we can do for ourselves.

Try using the metta phrases with old boyfriends and girlfriends, parents, difficult in-laws, siblings, ex-friends, neighbors, and other people in any relationship that creates tension inside. It's easier than you think. If you feel ashamed of how *you* behaved in the relationship, make a special effort to recognize that emotional pain. Shame, guilt, and remorse are the trickiest emotions to identify because we're continually dodging them inside. Remember that not a single emotion is outside the range of self-compassion. Bring kindness to yourself *because* of your difficult feelings. Thereafter, extend good will to the other half of the relationship.

It requires special skill to work with traumatic relationships that may include physical, sexual, or verbal abuse. Most important, make sure you're prepared—that you have the emotional resources for your journey and the necessary support of a therapist, friends, or family. Disturbing memories can overwhelm our best intentions. Will you know when your capacity for compassion is running low and you need either to refocus on yourself or to quit the practice altogether? You're pushing it too hard if you find yourself unable to sleep, emotionally numb, having difficulty concentrating, or feeling unusually fearful and isolating yourself. Go slow and be safe.

Compassion Fatigue

The result of extending ourselves too much to others is called "compassion fatigue." The term is actually a misnomer because compassion itself isn't fatiguing. Compassion fatigue is really "attachment fatigue." We wear ourselves out when we're attached to the *outcome* of our hard work, such as the success or recognition. Sure signs of compassion fatigue are (1) believing that you're indispensable and (2) feeling resentment toward those you're trying to help. Compassion fatigue feels bad, and it's not good for anyone. The antidote to compassion fatigue is *self-compassion*. When your emotional supplies are depleted, take a break and care for yourself in whatever way you can: physically, mentally, emotionally, relationally, or spiritually.

Another way to manage compassion fatigue is by cultivating *equanimity*. When you're caught by excessive attachment, see if you can untangle yourself by contemplating: "People are the owners of their deeds. It's their choice how they make themselves happy or free themselves from suffering." This is a traditional Buddhist saying to cultivate equanimity. It may sound like a prescription for indifference, but when you're trapped in compassion fatigue it's your ticket to emotional freedom.

Altruism and Your Well-Being

The psychologist Martin Seligman says that people seek happiness in three different ways: the Pleasant Life, the Engaging Life, and the Meaningful Life. Research has shown that pleasure contributes *less* to overall happiness than either being fully engaged in your life or having a meaningful life. Being "engaged" means knowing your strengths (such as your "signature strengths" from Chapter 5) and building them into your relationships and leisure activities. When you're good at a task, you can become completely absorbed in it—you enter the "flow"—which is a deeply satisfying experience. A "meaningful life" is one in which you use your strengths for the *greater good*—something larger than yourself. Altruistic pursuits and metta meditation fit into this latter category.

Would you like to know how you're constructing your own life? If so, you can take the Approaches to Happiness Questionnaire, a quick test developed by Chris Peterson at the University of Michigan (*www.authentichappiness.sas.upenn.edu/Default.aspx*).

Seligman and Peterson's categories should be considered guides, not prescriptions, for any given individual. For example, some well-meaning people have a tendency to deny themselves pleasure as they pursue the greater good, which can make them harsh and judgmental. Other individuals may need a little encouragement to extend themselves to others so they can enjoy the satisfaction of making a difference in someone's life. Even absorption in daily activities, though highly satisfying, is not universally desirable. Periods of confusion and doubt are necessary for us to grow. Use your understanding of these three approaches to bring balance and happiness into your life.

TAKING IT ON THE ROAD

Loving-kindness and compassion practice can easily be integrated into daily life. Every moment that you use a metta phrase, you're doing informal meditation. It takes only a second of your time.

Walking Meditation

A delightful way to take metta meditation on the road, quite literally, is walking meditation. Whether you walk in the city or the woods, your mind will usually be in the "default" mode, digesting the past (who said what to whom) or planning the future (your errands, your evening). Our minds are mostly critiquing the people and things we see around us. Instead, we can use these walks to develop loving-kindness and compassion.

TRY THIS: *Compassionate Walking*

Plan to walk for 10 minutes or longer, anywhere you like. Dedicate the time specifically to cultivating loving-kindness and compassion.

- Stand still for a moment and anchor your attention in your body. Be aware of yourself in the standing posture. Feel your body.

- Recall that every living being wants to live peacefully and happily. Connect with that deep wish: "Just as all beings wish to be happy and free from suffering, may I be happy and free from suffering."

- Begin walking. Note yourself moving through space in the upright position. Feel the sensations of your body, perhaps noting the pressure of your feet on the ground or the wind in your face. Keep your eyes softly focused and walk at a normal pace.

- After walking for a few minutes, repeat the loving-kindness phrases to yourself:

  May I be safe.
  May I be happy.
  May I be healthy.
  May I live with ease.

The phrases will keep your attention anchored in your body and start to evoke the attitude of loving-kindness. Try to synchronize the phrases with each step or with each breath. It may help to shorten the phrases to a single word: "safe, happy, healthy, ease" or "love, love, love, love."

- When your mind wanders, gently return to the phrases. If you find yourself hastening to your destination, slow down and refocus on your purpose.

- Do this with kindness, especially a feeling of gratitude toward your feet for supporting your entire body. Appreciate the marvel of walking.

- After a few minutes, expand loving-kindness to others. When someone catches your attention, say to yourself:

    May you and I be safe.
    May you and I be happy.
    May you and I be healthy.
    May you and I live with ease.

You also say "May *you* be safe ..." or just "safe ... happy ... healthy ... ease" or "love ... love ... love ... love." Don't try to include everyone; just do it one person at a time, keeping the attitude of loving-kindness alive.

- Eventually include all forms of life in the circle of your loving-kindness, for example, dogs, birds, insects, and plants.

- Allow yourself to *receive* any expressions of kindness that may come your way.

- At the end of the walking period, stand still for a moment and repeat "May all beings be happy and free from suffering" before you go on to your next activity.

Compassionate walking meditation is especially fitting for people who can't sit still very long and for people who are sitting all day in front of a computer and would like to get some exercise. A common question is "What should I do if I have to talk with someone?" Just let yourself become absorbed in the conversation and keep the wish percolating in the back of your mind: "May you be happy and free from suffering."

Your heart will be full of loving-kindness when the metta phrases revolve spontaneously through your mind. Then, when you meet someone, your words will align themselves with the phrases. For example, the silent mantra "May you be healthy" may be expressed as "I'm so sorry you had the flu last week." You'll not only be speaking kind words; you'll actually *feel* them.

Other Everyday Applications

Do you remember the story I related in Chapter 3 of my struggle to help my wife after hip surgery? I was rescued from this domestic dilemma by mindfulness and loving-kindness practice. As I struggled to put my wife's shoes on her swollen feet, I had a flash of awareness ("Wow, this situation is going downhill fast") and self-compassion ("May she and I be free from suffering"). The metta phrase was the extra boost I needed to extricate myself from trying too hard to help my wife, which allowed me to get some orange juice and return to his task in a more sympathetic frame of mind.

Metta practice can also penetrate into sleep or near-sleep states of consciousness. Usually I say the phrases before I fall asleep and when I wake up in the morning. This habit seems to have transformed the irritation I first felt as my wife yanked the blankets off the bed during her hot flashes. These days, as the covers suddenly disappear from my shoulders in the middle of the night, I find myself muttering something mildly sympathetic, like "Estrogen depletion sucks, doesn't it?" as I wave the sheets in the air and create a little breeze for her. That's a minor marital miracle.

It's always good to keep some mindfulness meditation in your loving-kindness practice. That will keep you in your body when you feel bad, without trying to change anything, as Darlene discovered.

Darlene had a partner, Jackie, who suffered from mild depression. Jackie took care of their two kids while Darlene worked from her home office. Whenever Darlene went into the office, Jackie felt abandoned. Darlene felt guilty about this, and her stress came out as stomach pain and diarrhea. Over time, Darlene secluded herself more and more in her office. When Darlene finally discussed her problem with Jackie, Jackie reassured Darlene that she should go ahead and do her job even if she felt guilty about it. The ball was back in Darlene's court.

Darlene decided to approach the problem with mindfulness and self-compassion. First she resolved to find her emotions in her physical body rather than getting caught up in them—guilt, frustration, anger. She learned to recognize mild muscle tension in her gut and practiced "soften, allow, and love" (see Chapter 3). She labeled "guilt" in a soft, gentle way and recognized it as the same feeling she had as a child when her mother became disabled with migraine headaches. As Darlene reflected on her lifetime of guilty feelings, sympathy arose for herself. Rather than having a pity party, Darlene gave herself love: "May I be safe, may I be happy, may I be strong, may I live my life with ease." Then she added her beloved partner to the mix: "May *Jackie* be safe, may she be strong, may she be healthy, may she live with ease." "May *we* be healthy and strong, may we be free from suffering, may we live our lives with ease."

Whenever Darlene felt guilt, she located it in her body and resumed using the phrases. This practice put her in a good mood, and she started leaving the office for brief breaks with Jackie. Darlene had escaped her cycle of guilt, frustration, and avoidance, and Jackie's mood improved considerably. Changes such as these are likely to occur over just a few weeks. Mindfulness helps to keep metta practice grounded in moment-to-moment reality, and compassion softens the criticism we heap on ourselves and others when things go wrong.

As your practice gets stronger, you may want to bring the metta phrases into more challenging situations. For example, if you're having a problem with a noisy neighbor in the apartment upstairs, start by offering metta to yourself: "May *I* be safe, may I be free of bitterness, may I live with ease." Then include your neighbor: "May *she and I* be safe, may she and I be at ease." Then, "May *we* both be at ease, may we both be free from bad feelings, may we both figure out how to communicate with each other."

Be flexible in your use of metta phrases in daily life, customizing them for each situation. (In formal sitting meditation, it's better to keep the phrases the same.) Try not to make the phrases so specific that you get hooked on an outcome, such as "May she shut off the music already!" Of course, timely action is sometimes a more skillful approach than silent meditation, but in the long run the most effective interventions occur when we approach others with good will.

The Power of Compassion

Over the years, I've learned to trust the power of compassion to heal relationships. The following incident, which occurred during a couple therapy session, reinforced that trust:

Jim worked conscientiously as a photographer but never seemed to earn enough money. Ruth was in despair about this, and occasionally she flew into a rage. This happened once during a therapy session. Ruth just seemed to snap, calling her husband a poor provider, "half a man," and "lazy." The words were so harsh that they felt surreal to me, like watching a made-for-TV movie about marital conflict. Jim remained calm throughout the tirade and intently focused on Ruth, which I found both curious and comforting. When it was over and I asked Jim what was going through his mind, he replied, "As the poison was coming out of Ruth's mouth, all I could see was the pain in her heart."

The following session, I learned that Ruth had grown up under difficult economic conditions and she was terrified of returning to that lifestyle. When this issue came out into the open rather than remaining a hidden terror in Ruth's heart, the couple was able to candidly discuss their financial needs and brainstorm together about the future. Ruth even volunteered to take over the financial side of Jim's photography business, which Jim gratefully accepted.

This outcome would have been impossible without Jim's deep compassion—it made space for a deeper conversation about the soft feelings behind the hard words. Everyone in an intimate relationship occasionally leads their pain with fighting words. Jim's remarkable comment "As the poison was coming out of [her] mouth, all I could see was the pain in her heart" has become an anchor for me when I'm with couples in intense conflict. Happily, Jim's business is now flourishing, thanks to Ruth's skillful guidance.

Another surprising experience I had as a psychotherapist was an instance of compassion:

Sam arrived in my office looking tense and distracted. He had just called for an emergency consultation a number of years after I'd last seen him. Within a few minutes, Sam blurted it out: "I have to help my mother kill herself and I'm here because maybe you can help me." I was shocked and perplexed. I'd been a therapist for over 15 years and had never had such a request, especially not from a reasonable guy like Sam.

It all made sense when Sam began to explain. His mother had suffered a stroke, and she couldn't speak, eat, walk, or toilet herself. Sam said he could read in her anguished eyes that she was begging him to end her life. Knowing a little about strokes, and buying some time as well, I suggested to Sam that he should probably wait before taking drastic action because his mother might recover some functioning over the coming year.

I never heard from Sam again on this issue. When he called for an appointment a year later to discuss a different problem, I asked him how his mother was doing. He said, "Oh, she's much better." I inquired what that meant, and Sam said she had not recovered any physical capacity, but she seemed happier than she'd ever been in her whole life. "How could that be?" I wondered aloud. Sam explained that his mother was always the kind of person who was supercompetent, never let others do anything for her, criticized his father mercilessly their entire life together, and now his dad was happily taking care of his mother in every possible way. "My mother was forced to receive love, perhaps for the first time in her entire life," Sam said, "and it seems to have made her a gentler person."

Uncommon kindness, combined with curiously favorable conditions, seems to have created this remarkable outcome.

A final example of the power of loving-kindness and compassion concerns my dear friend from graduate school, Gib, and his wife, Faye. Gib was 48 years old when he married Faye, then 32 years old, after the breakup of his first marriage. Faye had blond hair and drove a red convertible sports car with the license plate "FUN4-FAYE." Three years after they married, Gib was diagnosed with acute lymphoblastic leukemia, and the chemotherapy paralyzed him from the chest down. Faye remembers driving home after hearing the awful news, sobbing, "My husband is paralyzed! ... My husband is paralyzed! I don't want my husband to be paralyzed!" When I visited Faye and Gib 2 years later, I asked Faye, "How do you do it?" Her response has echoed in my mind ever since. She softly replied, "I didn't know I could love so much."

"It's been a process," Faye told me. "We've had good counselors and ministers. And Gib allows me to talk. Most of the time he's a husband and not paraplegic. He allows me to be me because of who he is." Faye added, "I don't see that blond bombshell anymore, but Gib can see the beauty of my soul. God has called us to love on a soul-to-soul level. He stripped away much of what we had together initially, forcing us into a deeper level of understanding of each other. The love we have now is nothing short of a miracle."

Eight years ago, a bright light entered Faye and Gib's life in the form of an adopted daughter. When their daughter started school, Faye returned to her work as a school teacher. At one point, Faye started worrying about herself: "When parents tear up, I tear up with them. I do the same with just about anybody." Then someone told Faye, "That's not weak, that's compassion!"

I hope this chapter has helped you learn how to integrate loving-kindness practice into your life, without losing yourself. In Part III, I'll show you how to tailor self-compassion to your personality style and circumstances, how to sustain your practice over time, and how to gauge your progress.

Part III

customizing
self-compassion

8

finding your balance

Man always travels along precipices, and, whether he
will or no,
his truest obligation is to keep his balance.
— José Ortega y Gasset, *Spanish philosopher*

The next step is to customize your self-compassion practice. A
key element is to balance your personality style—how you
typically deal with stress—so self-compassion can unfold naturally in your life. For example, a "caregiver" personality might easily feel compassion toward others but hold back on self-compassion.
An "intellectual" may understand the concept of self-compassion
but find it difficult to get on board with the emotional aspect. A
"butterfly" can be enthusiastic about self-compassion practice at
first, but fly away at the first sign of difficulty. By knowing how
you're built, you can make the most of your strengths and minimize
obstacles that will invariably crop up.

There are also challenges that arise for *all* types of people while
doing self-compassion practice. These are known as the "hindrances"
in Buddhist psychology: *grasping, aversion, weariness, agitation,* and
doubt. It helps to know when you're caught in one of these mind
states. You may be skeptical, for example, about whether a person
who grew up in your family could ever develop self-compassion—

that's "doubt." Or you may want to experience the fruits of the practice *immediately*—that's "grasping." Being able to name and work with the hindrances will make the practice go a lot more smoothly. Taken together, knowing your personality style and what's hindering you from moment to moment can save you a heap of trouble.

BEING THERE NOW

When I first learned to meditate in 1976, I felt the most important thing in life was to become spiritually enlightened. I meditated with a vengeance, occasionally becoming quite anxious and irritable. After a few months, I realized I was learning a lot about the mind—not a bad idea for an aspiring psychologist—but I was becoming rather unpleasant to be with. Then I thought, "What's the point? Why suffer now for rewards in the distant future? Isn't it a better idea to cultivate well-being gradually, every moment of the day?" Kindness is both the means to and the end of practice. These days, when I find myself struggling too hard at meditation, I simply repeat the metta phrases "May I be happy, may I live with ease." That immediately softens my body and mind. Your own meditation practice will be in balance when you experience the four cornerstones of loving-kindness—safety, happiness, health, and ease—in this very moment. That's the goal.

The beauty of self-compassion practice is that you don't need to look far to see if you're on the right track. Are you meeting your daily experiences with kindness? Regardless of whether you're meditating, putting your kids to bed, or stuck in a traffic jam, the question is "how" you're doing it. *Do you have good will toward yourself or not?* It's that simple. And when you detect discomfort—perhaps struggling for something you want or trying to avoid what you don't want—can you feel compassion toward yourself and soften into the experience?

The expectation of well-being is your best teacher. Then, when safety, happiness, health, and ease are *not* happening, you'll be alerted.

Pay attention to the experience of discomfort. Then decide what to do. Should you focus on the breath to calm your mind? If you feel tense and contracted, should you open your awareness to other sensations? Should you just give yourself love? These options arise more easily when you have a standard of well-being with which to evaluate your mental condition.

When you experience the same kind of distress over and over—body tension, doubt, loneliness—it becomes time to examine your personality style. Are you striving too hard? Do you expect perfection? Are you lonely because you're using meditation to avoid social contact? Although uneasiness is a natural occurrence in meditation, prolonged distress is a wake-up call to look at your invisible frame of reference: your personality. We all need to go there from time to time.

WHAT PERSONALITY TYPE ARE YOU?

Our personalities are the containers for our attitudes, thoughts, feelings, and actions. They are what we call the individual "self." Without your personality, you wouldn't be you! The job of a meditation teacher is to work with each unique personality and find a way to make the practice happier and more fruitful. Usually that requires softening certain aspects of who we think we are. Knowing your personality style can help you become your own best teacher.

The following 12 personality styles are offered as aids to practice. They are anecdotal rather than scientifically derived. I could have used one of the existing personality typologies (such as the popular Myers–Briggs Type Indicator), but none of those measures speak directly to the kinds of challenges that appear during self-compassion practice. You may see yourself in one or more of the following personality styles. Feel free to make a category of your own if you can't identify with any of them.

Our personalities are built primarily around the need to survive rather than to be happy, so rest assured that some aspects of your personality will run counter to emotional well-being and the practice of self-kindness. Try to identify the personality styles that predominate in your own life and examine their impact on your practice.

As you review these categories, let yourself be good-natured about it. Nobody's perfect. We all need conditioned ways of being in the world—we need a "self"—so we don't have to reinvent ourselves every moment of our lives. But what worked for you as a child may not work so well when you're an adult, and what works when you're with your lover may not work when you're trying to bargain down the price of a new car. The purpose of this chapter is not to change or critique your personality, but rather to *balance* the effect it might have on your self-compassion practice. Start by assuming that we're continually slipping in and out of balance as we juggle the demands of daily life.

Caregiver

Does extending compassion to yourself immediately make you think of someone else who needs it more than you do? Caregivers find meaning in life by caring for others. They're likely to thrive as a parent, nurse, or counselor. (The intrinsic satisfaction derived from helping others may compensate somewhat for the relative lack of monetary rewards in caregiving professions.) Women are more likely than men to be caregivers. Caregivers are good at compassion—accompanying another person, emotionally and physically, through periods of hardship and distress.

The main threat to the happiness of caregivers is attachment to the outcome of their labors. They find it hard to give love and not control how things will work out. I heard of one "helicopter parent" who went with her son to his first job interview after college and questioned the interviewer afterward about her son's interviewing skills! Caregivers can also lose their peace of mind when they overidentify with the suffering of their loved ones, as reflected in the saying "A mother can only be as happy as her *least happy* child."

Being compassionate with oneself is an effective balm for vicarious suffering, but caregivers often feel they're *abandoning* their loved ones if they attend to themselves. Taken to an extreme, a caregiver may feel that she's not a "caring person" if she isn't struggling at the edge of her capacity. The thought is "If I worry enough, my son will be safe!" Some mothers find self-compassion comes more easily when they say, "Just as I wish that my daughter be safe and happy, so may I be safe and happy." That comforts both sides of the worry equation—both subject and object—in the caregiver's mind.

Caregivers may also deny their own suffering by saying "Yes, but he has it *so much worse than I do*." Minimizing one's own pain by comparing it to others interferes with self-compassion because we have to feel our pain in order to evoke compassion. How do we love others without losing ourselves? We start by practicing mindfulness of our own discomfort ("This hurts!"). Then we soften into the physical feelings and treat ourselves kindly in both word ("I love you!") and deed (for example, a warm bath, a walk along a river). Embracing ourselves during hard times protects us from fatigue and resentment and gives us the energy to be present for others.

Intellectual

Does self-compassion practice seem too touchy-feely, requiring you to take leave of your mind? Intellectually inclined people use their rational minds to regulate emotions and solve problems. A fine example is the Dalai Lama, who recommends that we think about pain and suffering in the following way: "If there is a method of overcoming suffering or an opportunity to do so, you have no need to worry. If there is absolutely nothing you can do about it, worrying cannot help you at all." Such clarity of thought can be a comfort to more emotionally reactive people, especially in times of crisis.

But intellectuals can get out of balance through too much thinking (the Dalai Lama excluded!). Lama Surya Das says, "The intellect is a good servant but a poor master." When intellectuals are upset, they take the elevator to the top floor and can get stuck in their heads. Rational thought is an intellectual's most reliable means of solving problems, but sometimes the problem must be handled lower down. For example, traumatic memories are often locked in the body, and the body needs to be soothed to release them. Obsessing can provide short-term relief from emotional pain—it's a kind of escape—but it can also keep emotional problems simmering for a long, long time.

I've known a few intellectuals who never feel quite comfortable with loving-kindness practice. The phrases, such as "May I be safe," didn't seem credible. "*Safe,* you say? We're all going to die, so *no one is safe!*" It's especially difficult for the intellectual to grasp the difference between *wishing* and the *object* of wishing. Wishing is experienced in the chest region, not the head. It's an attitude that we feel rather than a thought process. Fortunately, the sense of simply wishing, without being bound to the object of the wish (health, happiness), can be experienced by anyone after sufficient practice.

Some intellectuals recognize the value of self-compassion practice when they're in dire distress—when thinking has not helped them escape their predicament. Even the most intellectual person is a sucker for love when he or she feels terrible. That's when the intellectual settles for "care," rather than "cure." Other intellectuals develop a gradual appreciation of self-compassion through mindfulness practice. They discover that they need to add loving-kindness to the mix when confronted with deeply disturbing feelings or else they can't think at all.

Intellectuals are also likely to have a problem with the notion of "self" in self-compassion. "Aren't we reinforcing a fiction," they ask, "that makes us feel even more separate and lonely? Isn't it better to focus on moment-to-moment experience as it arises, without superimposing a 'self'?" This point of view is entirely correct when we're feeling good. When the sense of "self" is in pain, however, the healthiest response is to go where the pain is located. Our attention will automatically move beyond the limited "self" when disturbing emotions have subsided.

Perfectionist

Are you frustrated by how un-self-compassionate you are, or by the stubbornness of old emotional habits? Perfectionists reap the benefits of high standards, but they continually fall short of their own expectations. When is "good enough" good enough? Probably when you're younger, prettier, smarter, richer, stronger, healthier, and happier. The self-help industry is based on the cultural assumption that we're never good enough. Women, in particular, are assaulted on all fronts by their supposed inadequacies.

Perfectionism begins in childhood. If a parent has excessively high standards for giving approval, the child can carry a sense of inadequacy long into adulthood. Alternatively, if there were *no* standards and the parent was emotionally distant, the child may develop unrealistic standards for him- or herself about what is required to receive love.

The main difficulty perfectionists have with self-compassion practice is their relentless need to improve: "I must be doing this wrong!" Remember that meditation is an even playing field; the only "experts" are those who are willing to return again and again to the practice. You'll *never* meditate properly or be sufficiently self-compassionate, but you'll also never fail as long as you stick with it. One extra moment of self-kindness during the day is enough. Criticizing yourself is the opposite of self-compassion. I've found that perfectionists become the most ardent practitioners of self-compassion once they break out of the self-improvement trap.

The only prerequisite for receiving compassion is suffering, and perfectionists suffer all the time from feelings of inadequacy. Perfectionists can start the practice right there, in the pain of never measuring up. Perfectionists can also balance their tendency to criticize themselves by *forgiving* themselves for their shortcomings, by training themselves to feel *gratitude,* and by *savoring* positive experiences (see Chapter 5). Those are all learnable skills.

Individualist

Is it uncomfortable to explore your feelings when things go wrong or to share them with others? Individualists prefer to be independent and to conduct their lives without interference from others. They don't expect to be helped when they're in trouble, nor do they feel obligated to help others. "Each person is responsible for his or her own destiny," they say. Individualists don't need or want anyone's pity.

Individualists are attractive to people who admire self-reliance. They take on seemingly insurmountable challenges without complaining. Since individualists don't actively seek out comfort and support, they can secretly feel lonely or unappreciated when their efforts aren't recognized. Loved ones often struggle to feel close to individualists and may eventually give up trying.

Individualists need to be strong and in control. I've known some individualists who take up self-compassion practice specifically so they won't need to rely on other people. This doesn't usually work because there's a limit to how much we can let go internally if we think there's no one to assist us in times of need. Many people have told me they wept after a loved one died only while in the company of others. If you're an individualist, reflect on the people who rely on you and who might be *honored* to help you if you needed it. You might be less alone than you think.

Softening in response to pain is a foreign concept to the individualist. If you're an individualist, remember that it's not a sign of weakness to feel the gravity of your own struggle. Even the toughest characters can be broken-hearted and need support. There's always another day to soldier on.

Survivor

Do you feel you don't deserve love and attention? Survivors suffer from what a pioneer in the field of self-compassion, Tara Brach, calls the "trance of unworthiness"; they don't trust the validity of their own feelings or feel entitled to feel good. Some survivors have been neglected or abused as children and are struggling to create a life worth living. Survivors are often soulful individuals on a lifelong quest for deeper meaning. They can be quite compassionate toward others who suffer harm and injustice, acutely aware of the cruelty and suffering that people inflict on one another.

Many of the challenges that survivors face on the path to self-compassion have been mentioned earlier. Self-criticism is a common consequence of years of neglect or abuse ("I felt bad; therefore I *am* bad"), which can make it difficult to even start self-compassion practice. It's obviously quite difficult to extend love to yourself if your mother said, "I wish I had never taken you home from the hospital." An open heart can also cause "backdraft": a burst of repressed memories. These memories can be intense and unpredictable, overwhelming our awareness. To make matters even worse, the survivor may shut down emotionally when feeling good, instinctively fearing punishment for not suffering. Love can be both unfamiliar and dangerous to the survivor.

Nevertheless, a therapeutic dose of self-compassion is balm for a survivor. Compassion is ready to flow because pain is a constant element in the life of a survivor, but it helps to first direct it toward *others,* especially a child or a pet. The survivor can eventually redirect kindness back to herself—tuck herself into the circle of love—in a safe and timely manner.

Workhorse

You can't find time for self-compassion practice? "Work" refers to what we do for extrinsic goals, like money, power, or fame; "play" refers to what we do for its own sake, like enjoying flowers or reading a novel. On rare occasions, work *is* play: Confucius said, "Choose a job you love and you will never have to work a day in your life." Self-compassion practice should be understood as a time to enjoy being yourself—more like play than work.

Americans are a culture of workhorses. Twice as many Americans as Europeans work more than 50 hours a week. In our spare time, we try to improve ourselves as well—the self-improvement industry is worth over $9.6 billion annually. Workhorses plan every minute, multitask, and feel annoyed when their schedules are interrupted. They generally overwork despite the cost to their health and relationships.

The main challenge to a workhorse is stopping or slowing down. There's never a good time for the workhorse to practice self-compassion, either formally or informally. When time allows, other goal-directed activities will immediately take priority: replying to an e-mail, catching up on world events, doing the laundry. Meditation is about "being." Workhorses will turn "being" into "doing"—they will stress themselves while doing loving-kindness meditation.

The workhorse needs to get off the treadmill just long enough to feel the stress of the time-intensive lifestyle. Such moments come to everyone, perhaps on the occasion of one's 50th birthday, when the doctor says it's time to start blood pressure medication, or after a heated argument with an inconvenient teenage son. Mindfulness of "urgency"—the feeling of toppling forward—can be the first step toward reestablishing balance. Then we apply loving awareness to the difficult emotions that arise during quiet contemplation, perhaps feelings of anxiety, loneliness, or fear of dying. Self-compassion is a relatively safe way to meet these demons lurking in the heart of the workhorse.

The workhorse will try to achieve the goal of freedom from suffering in record time. Once the workhorse has begun to practice self-compassion, he or she should guard against becoming overly zealous about it. The workhorse needs to find a healthy balance between striving and leisure.

Butterfly

Will you likely grow tired of self-compassion practice soon after starting? Butterflies are charming, enthusiastic people who become easily engaged in new ideas. They're delightful company because they devote their full attention to the people and situations in which they find themselves.

Consistency can be a problem for butterflies. They have difficulty seeing a project through to completion and keeping promises to themselves and others. Over the course of a lifetime, the butterfly may feel that he or she is continually starting over, making lateral moves in relationships, career, and residences. The butterfly is likely to skip from one meditation practice to another, like drilling for water 10 feet in 10 places, rather than 100 feet in one place. The butterfly sacrifices depth for breadth.

What does it take for a butterfly to stick with self-compassion practice? The butterfly first needs to experience the *cost* of flitting around: anxiety, loneliness, self-doubt. It's unrealistic to expect a butterfly to work exclusively with one practice (for example, using the same metta phrases), but understanding the underlying principles, like talking kindly to oneself, can keep the butterfly engaged in the practice for a long time while changing the specific techniques along the way. The support of like-minded individuals is another ingredient that helps the butterfly maintain a consistent practice. More will be said about sustaining a practice in the next chapter.

Outsider

Do you feel like you just don't fit in? Being an outsider in our society can become a core aspect of one's worldview. There are so many reasons to be marginalized by others: racial prejudice, homophobia, devaluation of women, invisibility of older people, insensitivity to poverty, religious intolerance, ethnic biases, and illness or disability. Is your family background at odds with your current living situation, perhaps because you're from a foreign country, a different socioeconomic class, or you had a difficult childhood? Even exceptional personal strengths like artistic ability or spiritual sensitivity can be invalidated by the dominant culture and make us feel like outsiders.

It's not necessarily bad to be an outsider. People living on the margins of society often have special insight into the unspoken assumptions of the majority. Martin Luther King said, "Almost always, the creative dedicated minority has made the world better." Compelling new music, writing, visual art, cutting-edge comedy, and social critique come from outside the mainstream. Besides, our materialistic cultural values are certainly not a prescription for happiness.

Nonetheless, the experience of disconnection from our culture can undermine one's basic sense of wholeness. Consider the metaphor of a fish swimming in water: as the fish lives and breathes, it draws water through its own body. We're like fish in the water of our culture, and when the water is polluted with racism, sexism, and ageism, we draw those prejudices inside. It's very difficult to be gay in a homophobic society without experiencing internalized homophobia, or Asian in a Caucasian culture without carrying around anti-Asian stereotypes. Self-image is inseparable from the culture that creates it.

Socially and culturally generated pain must be recognized and held in kindly awareness. Responding with bitterness to messages of fear, anger, or hatred increases suffering, as does prejudice silently taking root within us. Simply feeling invisible to the outside world can cause tremendous pain. The Ecuadorian essayist Juan Montalvo wrote, "There is nothing harder than the softness of indifference." If you feel like an outsider, start by noticing when you feel the pain and then respond to it with self-compassion: "May I be free from anger and fear." "May I love myself, just as I am."

Floater

Are you good at going with the flow and living in the moment? Floaters are generally agreeable people. They follow the tide and fit easily into new situations. They respect the opinions of others because every point of view is valid within a particular context. Their lives are directed more by synchronicity—seemingly random events coming together—than by personal goals and desires. They live in the present moment.

Taken to an extreme, floaters can be detached and noncommittal. For some floaters, "going with the flow" is an excuse for avoiding difficult challenges, resulting in passivity and lack of direction. The floater can become derailed during self-compassion practice when old emotional wounds surface.

The greatest challenge to a floater is *commitment*: identifying, trusting, and pursuing one's deepest convictions. The floater should begin self-compassion practice by asking, "What's my heart's desire? What really matters in my life?" Deeply held values and commitments (for example, relationships, work, health, leisure) help us overcome obstacles along the way. For example, the pain of childbirth is easier if a woman desperately wants to be a mother, and a bad job is tolerable when you really need the money.

Cultivating self-compassion requires commitment because it goes against the tide—the tendency to resist emotional discomfort and blame ourselves when things go wrong. Given that the floater is already skilled at present-moment awareness and letting go, self-compassion practice can be smooth sailing once the goal is firmly established.

Moralist

Do you become easily indignant with people when they behave badly? Moralists have a strong sense of right and wrong. They thrive in a parent role, such as law enforcement or clergy, where correct conduct and thinking are valued. Moralists can be relied upon to set clear standards and defend them against threat. The moralist attitude is often welcomed in times of political and social upheaval.

Moralists apply strict moral codes to themselves as well as to others. They're often surprised when they realize that other people's lives are conducted on an entirely different basis from their own. The poet George Herbert wrote, "Half the world knows not how the other half lives." Moralists can get caught in "righteous indignation" when they perceive an ethical lapse in others and can become excessively self-critical when they detect their own shortcomings.

During self-compassion practice, it's necessary for moralists to let go of preoccupation with how *other* people behave just long enough to discover how righteous indignation feels in their own bodies. The alternative to righteous indignation is not immorality but rather an assessment of what's necessary to guide others into less harmful activities. A more benign standard of behavior than "right" versus "wrong" is whether an action decreases or increases suffering. We don't need to stiffen ourselves in the presence of misbehavior to respond effectively.

A rigid ethical system also blinds us to unattractive parts of ourselves, such as lust, envy, greed, hatred, and selfishness, which makes them less manageable. We're repeatedly assailed by news reports of holier-than-thou politicians who get caught in sexual imbroglios. When we learn to recognize these all-too-human tendencies in ourselves, without shame and denial, we have a chance to steer them in more beneficial directions.

Finally, the moralist is likely to feel that self-compassion is self-indulgent. The self-indulgence argument can also be a way of dodging the unlovely aspects of our own personalities: what we don't know can't hurt us. Unpleasant feelings like lust, anger, envy, and greed will definitely pop up in the course of self-compassion practice, and hopefully the moralist can suspend self-judgment long enough to work with them.

Extravert and Introvert

Do you enjoy your own inner life, or do you prefer to be around others? "Extraverts" are gregarious, generally happy people who prefer the company of others rather than being by themselves. They enjoy activities like acting, political organizing, social networking, and management. They tend to think on their feet. Extraverts become restless when alone and are relatively unaware of psychological needs and problems.

In contrast, "introverts" enjoy the inner life. They like relatively solitary professions such as writing, art, and science. Introverts tire easily in social gatherings because they become overstimulated. Introverts are not necessarily shy—afraid of being criticized by others—but simply prefer their own company. They like to mull over what they plan to say before they speak. Research shows that genetic and brain differences may partially account for the differences in temperament between introverts and extraverts.

It would appear that extraverts are ill-suited for contemplative practices like meditation. Most of us, however, fall somewhere along a continuum from introversion to extraversion—we like good company and we appreciate periods of solitude as well. Self-compassion practice, especially metta meditation, has something to offer both introverts and extraverts because it is both solitary *and* relational.

There are a number of ways to adapt self-compassion practice.

The main challenge to *extraverts* is the uneasiness that can develop when sitting alone. The extravert should be encouraged to practice informally—during the day, while in the company of others—rather than tied to one place. For example, walking metta meditation (Chapter 7) fosters a sense of connection to others. When working with the loving-kindness phrases, the extravert can also emphasize the word "we" rather than "I" to feel connected with others ("May *we* be happy and free from suffering"). If you're an extravert and want to do sitting meditation, it's helpful to address uncomfortable feelings by labeling them as they arise ("bored," "restless," "anxious"). Finally, the extravert might enjoy the "Giving and Taking" meditation described in Appendix B. Giving and taking meditation is usually practiced in relationship to others, in both private and social settings, and it doesn't require as much psychological mindedness as metta meditation.

The challenge of loving-kindness meditation to *introverts* is just the opposite: it's often too relational, and the introvert needs to regulate just how much "relationship" feels comfortable. Since private meditation tends to come easily to introverts, they should be wary of using the practice to hide from social contact. Some introverts find that metta practice *reduces* their stress level in social settings when they send loving-kindness to the other people in the room. The goal for both introverts and extraverts is to maintain a healthy balance between solitude and engagement with others and to feel comfortable in both settings.

WHAT'S HOLDING YOU BACK?

Once you understand your personality style, you can also benefit from knowing the five mental "hindrances" that everyone encounters on the road to self-compassion: *grasping, aversion, weariness, agitation,* and *doubt.* Different people tend to be vulnerable to some of these traps more than others. For example, the caregiver tends to suffer from grasping, the moralist from aversion, the floater from weariness, the workhorse from agitation, and the intellectual from doubt. A hindrance may crop up at any time, and when we can identify it ("Ah, clinging"; "Oh yes, doubt"), it begins to subside. We don't want to battle the hindrances; rather, we want to accept their existence and work with them in skillful ways.

Start with the assumption that you *can* be free from suffering, in this very moment, right here, right now. Let a sense of well-being be the background of your practice. Then, when there's "disturbance in the field," ask yourself which of the following hindrances might be occurring. Bring mindfulness and loving-kindness to the hindrance, rather than trying to drive it out.

Grasping

We instinctively *grasp* for pleasure and for things that we hope will give us pleasure. If we don't get what we want, we feel disappointed. For example, imagine how you would feel if you discovered that your favorite musician would be playing in a nearby town, only to find out that the tickets were already sold out. A desire that hadn't even existed before leaves you feeling disappointed.

We also *cling* to what we enjoy and feel sad when it ends. If you had a nice bowl of ice cream, you might have wanted to enjoy the taste forever and felt disappointed when you finished it.

Grasping and clinging are similar expressions of *desire*. The Buddha said that desire is like taking out a loan; it's repaid by loss and separation when the pleasure is used up. Desire per se is not the problem; it's when we become a slave to our desires that we experience unhappiness. We need to hold our desires lightly.

We should be especially wary of becoming too attached to the good feelings that will arise during self-compassion practice. If you cling to love and happiness, your practice will become more frustrating than uplifting. Good feelings will arise and disappear as night follows day. An antidote to the hindrance of clinging to pleasurable feelings is to return to the practice of cultivating good will for yourself in spite of how you feel. When you're disappointed, exercise self-compassion *because* you feel disappointed.

Aversion

This book is primarily about overcoming aversion. Other words for aversion are "avoidance," "resistance," "entanglement," "disgust," and "resentment." Aversion is what we instinctively feel toward disturbing feelings. We can experience aversion toward an *internal state,* like anxiety or depression; toward an *external object,* like an open wound or spoiled food; toward *other people,* in the form of anger or fear; or toward *ourselves.* The Buddha called aversion a "sickness" because it ruins our health, and the antidote he prescribed was loving-kindness.

Aversion keeps us from seeing what's bothering us, from understanding it, and from working with it skillfully. When aversion is directed toward ourselves, we lose the ability to comfort and forgive ourselves for our mistakes. Sharon Salzberg suggests that we look at anger and aversion from the perspective of a Martian who's seeing them for the first time. "What is *this*?!" Curiosity is the first stage toward overcoming aversion. The subsequent stages, given in Chapter 1, are "tolerance," "allowing," and "friendship." We can move gradually from timid curiosity about what ails us to appreciation and respect. The same is true for the shameful and unlovely parts of ourselves. Self-kindness gives us the chance to learn more about what's bothering us, and ultimately to release it.

Weariness

This hindrance is also known as "dullness of mind," "mental inertia," "sloth," "torpor," and "boredom"—lack of interest in the practice of self-compassion. The opposite of weariness is the sense of delight that a child feels when encountering a fascinating object for the first time.

Is it possible to keep self-compassion practice as interesting as it felt in the beginning, perhaps with eyes moist with tears the first time you realized its true promise? That's unlikely, but it helps to remember *why* you started to practice. The reason was probably "to feel better!" Somewhere along the line you might have begun to practice in a mechanical fashion and forgotten your purpose. "I have to go to work ... got to meditate first ... can't concentrate ... 10 minutes to go. ..."

When you sit, see if you can really, REALLY, let yourself be happy and free from suffering. When discomfort arises, meet it with love and awareness and let it go. If you have a metta practice, savor the true meaning of the words and remind yourself of the target of the practice: yourself. Give yourself the experience of love and compassion however it comes most easily to you. Few of us can resist the attractive power of true love.

Weariness can descend upon the practitioner when the practice becomes too repetitive. The art of self-compassion, like all meditation, has an element of repetition. More than that, however, meditation is an active process of working with the skills of single-focus awareness, open-field awareness, and loving-kindness in creative sequences and combinations. Consider yourself like a captain on rough seas, always needing to make a course correction. Stay alert to the conditions that arise in each successive moment and make the most of them. You'll get bored and have a rougher ride if you switch to autopilot.

Agitation

Agitation is also known as "restlessness," "remorse," or "anxiety." It refers to dissatisfaction with the way things are and the need to move on ... somewhere, anywhere. The Buddha called agitation a tyrannical boss who's never satisfied. Regret over the past or worry about the future keeps the practitioner perpetually agitated.

Agitation can be quelled in numerous ways. The first step is to live your life with the fewest regrets. You'll feel the need to keep running if you leave a trail of misery behind you. Generous deeds can't protect you from being mistreated ("No good deed goes unpunished"), but you're more likely to feel peace of mind at the end of the day if you make others happy.

Another strategy for reducing restlessness is to appreciate the present moment. Ajahn Brahmavamso, a meditation teacher, said, "The fastest progress ... is achieved by those who are content with the stage they are on now. It is the deepening of that contentment that ripens into the next stage." How do we experience contentment in the present moment when the present moment doesn't feel good? Rather than daydreaming about the future, we can reanchor ourselves in the present moment by labeling exactly what we're feeling—"urgency," "restlessness," "anxiety"—and by softening into the physical experience of agitation. Restless legs? Clenched teeth? Deeper feelings may emerge when we don't react to restlessness, such as fear of being forgotten or left behind. Once we contact the discomfort of restlessness, or the suffering behind it, compassion can flow naturally. And the agitated heart will rest when it feels truly loved.

Doubt

The last hindrance, *doubt,* refers to skepticism about the practice or one's ability to succeed at it. When the mind is doubting, it isn't experiencing compassion or loving-kindness. Much time and energy are wasted in doubt.

The questions that most students bring to their meditation teachers are often tinged with doubt. For example, "Will I *really* make progress if just accept what I'm feeling in the present moment?" Teachers listen compassionately to their students' experiences, validate positive changes, and generally leave their students feeling less alone and more optimistic. The Buddha said doubt was like being lost in a desert. Every student will get lost from time to time in the particulars of his or her experience and will need someone or something that reveals the bigger picture. Buddhist psychology is such a roadmap and has been guiding students for over 2,500 years.

The student can also document his or her *own* progress to see if the practice is effective. Have you had moments of unexpected happiness since beginning self-compassion practice? Has your inner dialogue become more benign? Are you becoming more sympathetic to the plight of others? Have old relationship conflicts begun to ease up? The next chapter will go into the matter of "progress" in greater detail.

BRINGING IT ALL TOGETHER

The practice of mindfulness and self-compassion will gradually reshape your personality. That means that your usual ways of handling problems will become less automatic and you'll have the freedom to *choose* how to respond to a given situation. Other people may say that you've changed, but you may just be feeling more and more like yourself.

To recap, the first step toward inner transformation is mindful awareness that you're feeling emotional discomfort. The next step is self-compassion. That's mostly what's required to alleviate emotional suffering. With consistent practice, you'll develop a habit of sensing uneasiness in your emotional landscape and make shifts in attitude and attention without even being consciously aware of it. It's a new relationship with yourself that feels like having a loving companion by your side all day long.

FACE Your Challenges

There will always be times when conscious intention is required to deal with difficult emotions. The following four steps—F-A-C-E—can help you meet such challenges:

1. **F**eel the pain.
2. **A**ccept it.
3. **C**ompassionately respond.
4. **E**xpect skillful action.

Step 1, *feel the pain,* refers to mindfulness: knowing what you're experiencing *while* you're experiencing it. You can't work with pain if you're hiding from it. Mindfulness of pain means we actually *feel* it, not just keep it at a distance.

Step 2, *accept it,* means active, nonjudgmental embracing of experience in the here and now. Acceptance reverses the impulse to fight discomfort and thereby make it worse.

There are a host of ways to meet emotional difficulties with mindfulness (Step 1) and acceptance (Step 2). Some techniques emphasized in this book are *softening, allowing,* and *labeling,* described in Chapters 2 and 3. "Softening" refers to accepting the bodily manifestation of stress. "Allowing" means accepting the emotional experience of discomfort—letting it be just as it is, free to come and go. "Labeling," or naming how we feel, helps us disentangle from it.

Step 3, *compassionately respond,* means bearing witness to your own pain and responding with kindness and understanding. To do this, you can use the loving-kindness phrases or any of the other pathways to self-compassion mentioned in Chapter 5 or in Appendix B. The more we suffer, the more self-compassion we need, but sometimes that's the hardest step to remember.

Step 4, *expect skillful action,* means you'll be in the right mind-set to tackle even the trickiest dilemmas when you're mindful and compassionate. This could mean getting out of an abusive relationship, changing your job, or letting go of your resentment and accepting someone's shortcomings. Maybe you'll want to apologize to someone and ask for forgiveness. The behavioral options are unlimited.

Facing Back Pain, Insomnia, Stage Fright, and Difficult Relationships

The conditions described in Chapter 1 of this book have their root in resistance to emotional distress. For example, Mira herniated a disk while doing yoga. It hurt physically, but, more than that, it signified to her the end of her vigorous lifestyle. That was a shocking and unacceptable possibility for Mira, so she became obsessed with the problem, blamed herself for her misfortune, and reduced her level of physical exercise, which led to tighter muscles and increased pain. The healing path began after Mira learned how fighting her condition only made it worse. Her progress went from Step 1, feeling the pain rather than trying to resist it; to Step 2, accepting what was happening to her; to Step 3, not beating up on herself emotionally; to Step 4, intelligently caring for herself with massage therapy and moderate exercise.

Insomnia treatment follows a similar pathway, assuming you've ruled out physical and environmental causes of insomnia. Rather than ruminating all night long about the consequences of not sleeping, which can keep the nervous system on high alert, you need to recognize how much emotional distress you feel in the very moment of ruminating (Step 1). Then you accept your sleeplessness as a fight you can't win (Step 2) and respond with kindness (Step 3). One friend related the following incident when his wife had a cold and shifted about restlessly in bed beside him: "When I stopped wanting her to be more still, I started rubbing my head, got up to read a magazine, and, of course, quickly fell asleep in 5 minutes. If I kept 'griping,' I would have laid awake in bed for hours in frustrated resentment." His acceptance of the situation led to a self-compassionate response—rubbing his head—which eventually led to falling asleep.

If you still can't fall asleep when you accept your sleeplessness, it may be that the mind is troubled with overstimulating thoughts. You should then gently steer your attention to less energizing topics. One such exercise is simply to feel the sensation of each outbreath—mindfulness of breathing—and to recite a metta phrase with each exhalation. The loving-kindness phrases will take the edge off your struggle, and the boredom of repeating the mental exercise over and over will help you drift off to sleep, as long as you're practicing this exercise *for its own sake* and not keeping yourself on edge by doing it to fall asleep.

Managing stage fright follows a similar trajectory. Let yourself be anxious, feel it in your body, expect that fear is a natural human response to speaking to a large number of strangers, give yourself some love for being in that uncomfortable position, and then, perhaps, refocus on what you have to say. Dedicating yourself to benefiting your audience with a few good ideas removes the "self" that feels the worry.

Treating the Addictions

Self-compassion is no stranger to substance abuse treatment. When an Alcoholics Anonymous (AA) member says at a meeting, "I'm an alcoholic," he or she is speaking from a larger frame of self-acceptance—nothing to hide. Resisting the idea that one is an alcoholic, or becoming engulfed in shame when a relapse occurs, can be obstacles to staying clean and sober.

Alan Marlatt and colleagues at the University of Washington created a "mindfulness-based relapse prevention (MBRP)" program for alcohol and substance use disorders. It's an 8-week program that combines Jon Kabat-Zinn's mindfulness training with cognitive–behavioral techniques. Participants are taught about craving; they identify triggers for substance use—feeling, thoughts, and situations—and they learn to "urge surf." Key features of the MBRP program are accepting one's experience, seeing thoughts as just thoughts, taking care of oneself, and finding balance in life.

Another approach was developed by Kelly Avants, Arthur Margolin, and colleagues at Yale University School of Medicine: spiritual self-schema therapy (3-S⁺). It is intended for addiction and HIV-risk behavior in people of all faiths, although it's based in Buddhist psychology. In this 12-session, manual-guided program, participants learn to move from the addict schema ("addict self") to the schema of abstinence and harm prevention (the "spiritual self"). Metta meditation is taught in session 6 to increase awareness of harm caused by anger and hatred and to increase compassion. A research study designed by Zev Schuman-Olivier at Harvard Medical School showed that the 3-S⁺ program resulted in decreases in impulsivity and intoxicant use and greater motivation for abstinence compared to a standard care comparison group. One participant responded in the following way to a question about what she found helpful: "The meditation. That people deserve to be happy and free. My breathing, taking time out for myself, treating myself to something good sometimes."

Finally, difficult relationships necessitate that we drop first into our own emotional pain, validate what we're feeling, and then listen with kindness and understanding to what the other person has to say. We all have vulnerabilities that make us pull away from one another. In the episode described in Chapter 1 involving Michael and Suzanne, they witnessed how their vulnerabilities had pulled them apart (Michael pursuing his workaholic ways and Suzanne reacting with panic about their marriage), they felt the pain of disconnection from one another, accepted the pain as a sign of wanting to be closer, gave themselves credit for trying so hard to support the family, and learned to speak with one another in a less reactive, more positive manner: *I miss you!*

Mindful Self-Compassion Meditation

Sometimes we need a "time out" to disentangle from the automatic thoughts and feelings that rule our daily lives. I practice the following meditation in my own life, and I teach it to distraught clients in therapy. It takes only 5 minutes once you're familiar with it, and it synthesizes much of what you've already learned in this book. You can also stretch this meditation to 30–45 minutes, as you like.

TRY THIS: *Mindful Self-Compassion Meditation*

- Sit in a comfortable position, close your eyes, and take three deep relaxing breaths.

- Open your awareness to the sounds in your environment. Come into the present moment by simply listening to whatever presents itself to your ears.

- Form an image of yourself sitting in the chair. Note your posture as if you were seeing yourself from the outside.

- Next, bring your awareness *inside* your body. Note the world of sensation occurring there in this very moment.

- Now feel your breathing wherever it's most obvious to you. Pay special attention to every out-breath. (Use a different anchor for you attention if you feel more comfortable doing so.)

- Replace your out-breath with the loving-kindness phrases. For the next few minutes, slowly repeat the phrases, returning now and again to an image of yourself sitting in the chair.
- Gently open your eyes.

Facing Emotional Pain in Meditation

The following example illustrates how we can work in meditation with mindfulness and self-compassion to establish a new relationship with ourselves and the world in which we live.

Natasha is a single 32-year-old family physician who began practicing mindfulness meditation to help herself relax. She is the daughter of hardworking parents who desperately wanted her to become a successful doctor. Natasha learned to value achievement just as much as they did, which also meant she hardly found the time to socialize or unwind. It didn't really matter to Natasha until recently, when she discovered her friends were getting married and having children. Natasha just seemed to be getting tired.

Mindfulness meditation worked very nicely for Natasha at first, especially the calming effect of focusing on her breath for half an hour each morning and taking conscious breaths throughout the day. After a few months, however, Natasha noticed that focusing on her breath was making her anxious. She worried that breath meditation had stopped working for her, or worse. Sometimes Natasha found herself taking deep breaths—gasping for air—during her meditation.

Natasha consulted with her meditation teacher, who suggested that she was focusing too hard on her breath and she should open her awareness to other sensations that were occurring in the body. This helped, and Natasha discovered that her breath became a refuge again whenever she returned to it. She took the lesson to heart and broadened her informal practice to include the feeling of her feet on the floor. She especially liked this mindfulness exercise when appointments piled up near the end of the day and she was running from one examining room to another.

Natasha decided to go on a silent, weeklong retreat to deepen her practice. She chose a combination mindfulness/metta retreat. Natasha woke up at 5:15 A.M. and diligently attended every 40-minute meditation session for the first 3 days. Then she heard that teacher interviews were scheduled to begin on the fourth day. To her surprise, Natasha found herself stricken with fear about the interviews: "Will the teacher think I'm a good meditator? Will she like me?" Natasha meditated, hoping the fear would subside, but the more diligently she meditated, the worse it became.

Feeling broken and exhausted from fighting her fear, Natasha dragged herself to the meditation hall on the fourth morning. The morning meditation instructions were on loving-kindness meditation, especially metta for oneself. When Natasha sat down to practice metta meditation, it struck her like a revelation: "I don't have to concentrate, I don't have to be mindful, I don't need to apply more effort, I don't even need to calm down ... all I need to do is love myself because I'm in such a miserable state!" Natasha stopped using her breath as the anchor of her meditation and switched to the metta phrases. As she began ruminating about the upcoming interviews, she said to herself, "May I be safe. May I be free from fear. May I live my life with ease." Her body relaxed, and she found a tear trickling down her face. It no longer mattered what the teachers thought of her, or even what she thought of herself—she was okay just being who she was.

During the lunch break the same day, Natasha wondered to herself why she was so afraid of the interview. After all, the purpose of a meditation interview is to be supportive and helpful, not to judge. Natasha concluded that she was a perfectionist—self-critical and never good enough. She was the daughter of parents who desperately wanted her to be successful and financially secure. No matter how many A's she got on her report cards, her parents could never let up. Natasha internalized the message that she needed to strive relentlessly in order to prevent catastrophe.

Natasha decided it was time to live her life in a new way. She could hardly recall the last time she had taken a vacation. The dreaded interview eventually arrived, and Natasha shared with her teacher all that had occurred over the previous day. The teacher advised Natasha to cultivate a "preference for the present moment." The present moment is always a mini-vacation from striving—there are fewer worries because there's no future in the present. Natasha took this message to heart and started skipping sitting meditation sessions to walk in the woods, listen to the birds, and smell the earth. As she walked, she said to herself, "May I be safe. May I be happy. This moment, this *beautiful* moment."

When Natasha returned to her sitting meditation, she blended loving-kindness into her mindfulness practice. She used her breath to quiet her restless mind, she opened up to body sensations when she felt her breath shortening, and she used metta phrases when she felt disturbed or overwhelmed. Natasha learned to inhabit her body in a new, more loving, way.

During the remainder of the retreat, Natasha remained particularly vigilant to the hindrances of "clinging" (to calmness) and "aversion" (to fear). She recognized when she slipped into the "work-horse" or "perfectionist" mode. She labeled "striving" as it arose. Natasha also uncovered deeper feelings when she stopped striving— feelings of loneliness, fear, and emptiness—and she brought kindly awareness to these as well. Natasha had learned on her retreat to allow each moment to be just as it was—to simply sit.

Back at work, Natasha was surprised to notice how happy she was to see her patients and how carefully she listened to them. She had dropped an invisible layer of struggle—the struggle for approval—and she felt more at ease with others. Natasha also discovered she had more sympathy and understanding for her parents and the struggles they had gone through as she was being raised. She had found them in herself and knew the pain they unwittingly passed on to her. Natasha resolved not to transmit the same struggle for achievement to her own children, should she ever have the privilege of having kids.

Natasha's personal transformation might have eventually

occurred in daily life, but retreats can generate deep changes in a relatively short period of time due to the absence of ordinary distractions. In Natasha's case, she saw how her intolerance of feeling fear magnified anxiety into an intense situation. The only approach that helped Natasha was self-compassion. It opened her to further insights, such as underlying feelings of inadequacy and her fear of being left alone without anyone to rely upon if she faltered or failed. As Natasha validated herself with loving-kindness, her need for approval from other people began to subside. Natasha experienced a wholly unexpected sense of connection with others, including her patients and her parents. What had begun as an exercise in stress reduction evolved into a new, more compassionate way of life.

You now have the essential concepts and tools to cultivate self-compassion. The challenge, of course, is to practice them. There are so many pressing concerns and responsibilities in daily life that self-compassion is easy to forget. What does it take to maintain a practice over time? The next and final chapter will show you how.

9

making progress

Suffering doesn't disappear from our life, but into our
life.

—BARRY MAGID, *psychiatrist*

f you think it's hard to measure your progress on the path to self-
compassion, you're right. That's because the practice is paradoxical: we change by accepting ourselves more and more, bad feelings
and all. Since our usual standard for measuring progress is feeling
better, how do we know when we're on the right track? With self-
compassion, bad feelings can be a *good* sign—perhaps you're opening
up because you have the confidence and skill to handle them? Or
if you're frustrated by the tenacity of self-critical thoughts, maybe
you've finally become aware of your mental chatter? Or if you feel
that you're a hopeless case and have no self-compassion, perhaps it
reflects your growing *desire* to treat yourself well? This chapter will
explore what we mean by "progress" and offer suggestions for assur-
ing that progress is indeed made.

THE GRAND REFRAME

Self-compassion offers a novel approach to life experience: we sit
comfortably in the midst of our own uncomfortable emotions, let-

ting them take their course as we soothe and comfort ourselves. In the words of Ajahn Brahm, a meditation teacher, "When you visit someone in the hospital, talk to the person and leave the doctors and nurses to talk to the sickness." When applied to ourselves, that's self-compassion. We're attending to ourselves with great kindness, especially when our condition seems hopeless.

The key question is *"Am I meeting more and more of my life experience with kindness and understanding?"* That is, how *consistently* do you respond to yourself in a kindly way when things go wrong? Do you soothe and nurture yourself when you feel sadness, grief, longing, or rage? When you fail at something, are you sympathetic with yourself for failing? If you fall down 100 times, are you willing to pick yourself up 101 times? Is self-kindness gradually becoming a new way of life? A client of mine once remarked, "Taking 2 minutes more in a warm bath is one step toward staying in warmth one's entire life." Another said after a year of committed practice, "The practice is my own—now it works. I know the feeling. It's part of me."

You can't fail at this endeavor. Every day provides fresh opportunities to meet suffering with kindness, and every time you do that you're a success. Those moments may add up to a lifetime. You also have sufficient support for the practice—you were born with the motivation to be happy and free from suffering. The combination of innate desire and the self-rewarding nature of self-compassion will keep you on the path.

STAGES OF SELF-COMPASSION

Everybody starts practicing self-compassion in order to feel better. That's natural, but it's an ultimately flawed agenda because it pits us against the way things are, which leads to no good. Eventually we give up this agenda and move to a more refined understanding of the practice. Self-compassion goes through three distinct phases— *infatuation, disillusionment,* and *true acceptance*—culminating in self-compassion for its own sake.

Infatuation

I often introduce the loving-kindness phrases in therapy by saying: "If you feel comfortable doing so, please close your eyes, and I'd like to say a few phrases that you can roll around in your mind and carry with you throughout the week. They may make you feel better by changing how you treat yourself when things go wrong." Then I slowly recite the metta phrases two or three times: "May I be safe. May I be happy. May I be healthy. May I live with ease." People who've been fighting with themselves for a long time are attracted to the phrases like bees to honey. They fall in love with them. It's not uncommon for tears to flow if the practice is destined to make a significant change in the person's life. Tears signify the beginning of the end of the struggle.

One such person was Tanya, a 57-year-old magazine editor, who had been suffering for two decades from a severe case of insomnia. Previously, Tanya had given me three typed pages listing all the insomnia treatments she'd tried. She'd gotten to the point where she couldn't imagine living like that for another 30–40 years. I listened to Tanya's story for three sessions before she asked me to weigh in on it. I shared the loving-kindness phrases with her, and 1 day later Tanya wrote the following e-mail:

> I left your office yesterday with the phrases in my head. I dropped off the car at my husband's office, then walked along the Charles River to go home. The leaves on the trees and the grass were so green, almost neon, and undulating supernaturally. Everything seemed so vivid. I stopped to watch the goslings, then saw a seagull catch a fish. The air was almost a perfect temperature, though the light was dim through the heavy cloud cover. When I got home, I saw my new home from a different perspective. All of my hard work on it shone. The angles and curves of the architecture were apparent to me, as if I had just awoken to the beauty of it. I made dinner and enjoyed being in the house for the very first time. My husband came home and we had dinner and there was an easy tranquility between us. Then I went to bed ... and I slept almost the entire night. I just woke up twice.

Tanya's sleep improved dramatically for the next 5 weeks. Although an intense awakening like this is relatively rare, it reflects the sense of revelation that can occur when we let go and accept ourselves for the first time.

The infatuation phase of self-compassion eventually has to end, though, because it's based on the narrow wish to feel good. Like any love relationship, some unpleasantness eventually intrudes and pops the bubble of infatuation. But some important groundwork has been laid. The heady experience of loving oneself—letting go of fighting the way we are—gives confidence that seemingly intractable emotional problems can indeed be worked through.

Disillusionment

Disillusionment hits when the practice doesn't work anymore. It fits into a broader framework, succinctly stated by meditation teacher Rodney Smith: "All techniques are destined to fail!" That's because "techniques" are employed to feel better, and the only way to feel better in the long run is to abandon trying to feel better. Hence, all techniques are inherently flawed. More to the point, our underlying motivation is flawed, and it has to gradually shift if self-compassion exercises are to remain effective.

Although the disillusionment phase initially caused me some confusion, both as a practitioner and in my role as a psychotherapist, I have since learned to welcome it. Disillusionment is an opportunity as well as a crisis. For example, Tanya had a bad night after her first 5 weeks of refreshing sleep. She panicked and was up 14 times for 3 nights in succession. Her openness to giving herself kindness had been eclipsed by the older habit of trying to feel better. I reminded Tanya that trying so hard to fall asleep had caused 20 dreadful years of insomnia and we weren't going to allow her despair and panic to become the reason for another 20 years of this hell. The question was "Are you practicing self-compassion to fall asleep or *because* you suffer? It will fail if you use it to fall asleep, and it will succeed if you just love yourself when you are filled with fear and despair."

The disillusionment phase isn't fun. Tanya's struggle with disillusionment came out in another e-mail:

> But I feel angry ... at who or what, I'm not sure. I just feel very, very angry that I can't seem to rely on my body to sleep. It doesn't make me feel very optimistic about the future, and then I get even more angry. So okay, I will try not to try and just let it be.

The disillusionment phase is a "relapse" that can become a "prolapse"—a step forward—when we work with the problem behind the problem.

I often tell my patients in the disillusionment phase that the measure of their efforts is not how anxious or depressed they may feel from week to week, but how *willing* they are to feel that way. Acceptance is a more reliable measure of progress than random fluctuations in mood because it's the only factor that's under our conscious control. In Tanya's case, the questions were clear: How willing are you to be awake at night? Can self-compassion help you accept sleeplessness?

True Acceptance

True acceptance is a natural ripening of practice. It can't be forced. There's a wisdom aspect, plus the requisite kindness. When we truly accept, we realize in a deep, intuitive way that antagonizing ourselves is wasted effort and that the only intelligent alternative is to let go. In the true acceptance phase, acceptance and self-compassion can occur in a flash, often with only a touch of conscious awareness. One client of mine who formerly suffered from severe shyness hears himself saying whenever he gets a surge of anxiety: "Don't fight it!" The instinctive effort to avoid discomfort may linger somewhere in the background, but we've seen through it. We give ourselves kindness for its own sake.

True acceptance also has the experience of common humanity. We don't feel singled out by our personal idiosyncrasies. There's the sense that no matter what ails us, someone somewhere is probably struggling in the same way with the same dilemma. This was illustrated by Brenda (in Chapter 1), who said, "The pain of Zach's death has connected me to all mothers since the beginning of time who have lost children." The pain may be childhood trauma that predisposes one to fearfulness, or attention deficit disorder that makes it difficult to follow through on promises, or the social stigma of being too fat that makes us hide in shame. Whatever it is, we're not alone.

During the true acceptance phase, Tanya remembered that she had to look out for herself when she was a child because her mother was emotionally detached and her stepfather was scary and often cruel. In those days, Tanya stayed safe by remaining vigilant and invisible. It was taboo for her to have personal needs and dangerous to be seen because she could become a target for her stepfather's aggression. The adult Tanya still lived in fear of bad things happening to her. This insight—how she was programmed to fear, worry, and catastrophize—along with the recognition that she needed to nurture herself in a way that she had never learned as a child, helped Tanya drop some of her struggle with insomnia. She even began to see the value in welcoming sleeplessness because it was a prime opportunity to strengthen her new habit of self-compassion and because it helped her fall asleep.

The three stages of self-compassion—infatuation, disillusionment, and true acceptance—correspond to the phases of any good long-term relationship. First we connect with ourselves as we would connect with a new love. Then we discover that we're not protected from the pain of living and that we need to adjust to the conditions of our lives. Finally, we get to know ourselves very well and we accept what we can't change and acknowledge that we have to work skillfully with what we have. This evolution is a refinement of intention, moving away from always wanting things in a particular way to wisdom and letting go.

The stages also correspond to the shift from *cure* to *care*. In the infatuation stage, we have the underlying wish to cure what ails us. The disillusionment phase calls an abrupt halt to that agenda. In the true acceptance phase, we care for ourselves because life is hard and a merciful response seems the only intelligent option.

THE POWER OF COMMITMENT

Our intentions are subtle. We know from the research by Benjamin Libet described in Chapter 3 that our intentions are formulated in the brain even before we're aware of them and before we act. Neurologically speaking, the only option we have is to stop what's already under way, assuming we recognize early enough what's going on in our minds.

For our lives to go in the direction we want, it helps to reinforce those intentions and commitments that make the most sense to us. Usually we're on autopilot, following the hidden agendas of our genetically predisposed and conditioned personalities. For example, introverts may spend a lot of time avoiding people, caregivers might comfort themselves by helping others, and individualists may be secretly trying to get admiration for their intrepid self-reliance. These agendas take up most of our lives but may not be what we really want to do.

Psychologist Steven Hayes and colleagues have developed a model of psychotherapy based on core values and commitments. A good life is one in which we intentionally pursue what's most meaningful to us as we meet obstacles along the way with mindfulness and acceptance. What are your own core commitments? What do you want your life to stand for? What are your basic expectations in the areas of health, wealth, relationships, work, and spirituality? Do you primarily want your kids to be *happy* or do you want them to be *wealthy*? Do you want to live 100 years? What would you like to be said in your eulogy?

Perhaps you would like to take a moment and ponder these questions. Our commitments can be strengthened when we throw the force of conscious choice behind them.

One way to discover your intentions is to look at what you're already doing. What's the red thread that runs through your life? Are you choosing family over career? Do you like intellectual excitement more than physical thrills? Do you prefer social or solitary activities?

Most of us are at cross-purposes with ourselves. We value health, yet we run ourselves ragged at work. We treasure our families, but we lose patience with them every day. What do you *really* want? What's your heart's desire?

When you question yourself in this way, you may return to the innate wish to be happy and free from suffering. Not that our derivative commitments aren't essential for a valued life, but it helps to ask Why? *Why* do I want a happy family? *Why* do I want to stay healthy? Such inquiry takes courage, and the ultimate success of your self-compassion practice depends on how committed you are to being happy and well. If you haven't thought through your myriad responsibilities and commitments, you're less likely to benefit to the fullest extent from self-compassion practice.

How tightly should we cling to our core commitments? Hold them like a pen, not too tight and not too loose. Too tight causes cramping, and too loose will make the pen fall out of your hands. And don't be in a rush. The more deeply we settle into our experience, the more quickly our lives will change. Joseph Goldstein, one of the meditation teachers who started the Insight Meditation Society, suggests "relaxed persistence."

Also, try to make your commitments as pleasant as possible. We naturally avoid difficult activities. If it isn't pleasant, adjust it in some way. For example, don't think, "Now I have to meditate!" When you sit down for meditation, say to yourself, "The only thing I have to do now is be with myself as lovingly and happily as possible." Then use your skills—single-focus awareness, open-field awareness, and loving-kindness—to figure out how to do that. Let it be easy, even if it isn't.

MAINTAINING A MEDITATION PRACTICE

Many meditators have a dirty secret: they don't practice as much as they say. Trying to get a concrete answer to the question "How much do you meditate?" can be like asking for sexual secrets or how much money a person earns. I'm no stranger to this phenomenon either. If we ever meet and you ask this question, I hope I can respond humbly, truthfully, and with self-forgiveness. Forgiving ourselves when we fail to meet our own expectations is the first step toward sustaining a meditation practice. Some additional tips follow:

Shall I Sit?

Most people don't have a formal, sitting meditation practice. Why? Because most people don't feel very good when they close their eyes. Sooner or later (usually sooner!), we bump up against mental and physical discomfort. Why bother? The whole point of sitting meditation is to figure out how to be as happy as possible in our own skin. It helps to think of sitting meditation as a time to "be" without any other obligations and responsibilities, and go from there.

We don't need to do sitting meditation, but we need to *practice*. Practice means "systematic training by multiple repetitions." We're training the brain to function in a stronger, healthier way, just as an athlete trains the body. Donald Hebb, the father of neuropsychology, said "Neurons that fire together, wire together." Repetitive practice is essential. It needn't be boring, however: I'm pleased to report that although meditation is old and familiar, most days it still feels interesting to me because each moment is new—never came before, never to be repeated.

When and how you practice depends on your personal preferences and life circumstances. As I mentioned earlier, the easiest way to practice is *informally*: being aware whenever you feel emotional discomfort and responding with kindly awareness. Formal sitting meditation is more intensive practice, a chance to focus longer on the task at hand and to learn at a deeper level. The purpose of sitting, however, is to transform your daily life, not to get into altered states of consciousness. The most effective practice plan is to have both a formal (sitting) and an informal (daily life) practice to support each other. And whatever you decide to do, if it's not basically enjoyable, it's not self-compassion.

Start Small

Anyone can do sitting meditation—you just have to make it short enough. The simplest way to start the habit is to follow the "3-second rule"; *sit down for 3 seconds*. Who can't do that? If you previously had a practice and want to rejuvenate it, plan to sit down for a very short time. Three-second meditation overcomes the greatest barrier to practice: starting. Once you're sitting, it's easy to remain seated for longer periods.

Envision

If you want to meditate in the morning, start by envisioning the first 10 minutes of your day while you're still in bed. Will you go to the bathroom and then meditate? Will you go to the bathroom, have some tea, shower, and *then* meditate? If you can see the events unfold in your mind, you're less likely to be distracted by the rush of morning responsibilities. Similarly, if you meditate after work or before you go to bed, try to envision beforehand when and how you'll get to your meditation seat.

Make It Social

It helps to get together periodically with people who share your interest in meditation. If you don't have that opportunity, perhaps you can chat with sympathetic friends over the phone. You can also visit websites where meditators share their experiences, such as *yahoo.com/group/giftoflovingkindness*. Guided meditation tapes and related audiovisual materials can also provide a supportive context for practice.

Study

Our lives are usually driven by the cultural value of getting whatever we desire. Meditation teaches the opposite skill of wanting what we already have. Books written with wisdom and compassion are an invaluable aid to practice. They can be good companions on the path.

Find a Teacher

Having a teacher is an opportunity to learn from those who've gone before. A skilled teacher may be able to show how you're making the practice unnecessarily difficult, help peel away misunderstandings, remove doubts, and provide personal encouragement. Good teachers inspire as much by example as by what they say.

There still aren't many meditation teachers in the West, so it can be difficult to find a personal teacher in your geographic area. Most Western practitioners travel long distances to go on retreat and learn from a variety of teachers. Don't fret too much if you haven't found a personal teacher, though. A teacher is only as good as the student, and ultimately only you can transform yourself.

Go on Retreat

Retreats are an excellent place to learn the practice, to troubleshoot areas of difficulty, or to receive advanced training. They usually last from a few days to a few months. Most retreats occur in silence, except for daily meditation instructions, talks by teachers, and personal interviews. Silence alone has the effect of drawing out underlying emotional issues that we wouldn't recognize in daily life, which we learn to engage using the skills of meditation.

Two years ago, during meditation, I received a tap on the shoulder from the retreat manager, who told me with great tenderness that my father had just died. I left the retreat to see about funeral arrangements and to connect with my family, and when there was nothing further to take care of, I returned to the retreat. Sitting in the midst of my grief, occasionally weeping, smiling, regretting, and loving my father, I was reminded how healing it can be to have the company of compassionate people, even when they don't say a word.

FURTHER PRACTICE CONSIDERATIONS

Many questions will emerge as you progress on the mindful path to self-compassion. Questions are an important part of practice. A curious, welcoming attitude and a carefully framed question will create space in your mind for an answer to appear all on its own. You can learn to trust that. However, the following issues may have already arisen for you:

"My practice has done so much for me that I want to share the wealth. How can I get my family involved?"

It's generally best to keep your practice to yourself. Try not to become an annoyance to your loved ones by converting them to your practice. They'll be curious when they notice your good will toward them. Our nearest and dearest are definitely transformed by the practice ... when *we* change. They'll probably be living in a happier environment.

It's interesting, however, how naturally kids take to self-compassion practice. I received the following e-mail from the mother of a 2-year-old:

> We were driving back from southern Vermont, so Mia had been in the car seat for about an hour and a half already (pretty good for a 2-year-old) when we got stuck in traffic. At that point she'd had it with being in the car and car seat and she started to have a mini-meltdown. I started to say the loving-kindness phrases out loud, as a way of dealing with the terrible pain of watching my child in distress and not really being able to do anything about it. To my surprise (and extreme relief for both of us) the minute I started saying the phrases, she started responding to each phrase affirmatively and calmed right down. We got into a nice little cadence ...
>
> May we have peace in our hearts.
>
> Mia: Yeah.
>
> May we have joy in our hearts.
>
> Mia: Yes.

May we be free from suffering.

Mia: Okay.

May we live with ease.

Mia: Yes.

This went on for a couple of minutes, and then she was fine. I was especially surprised because I had already tried to soothe her by singing songs and by reaching into the back seat and playing with her.

Here's another thing I've noticed: sometimes when she is having trouble settling down for her nap I will say the phrases to myself, and it is as if the energy in the room changes, and she senses it and she settles right down.

Self-compassion may come easily to young children because they have not yet been tainted by social conditioning—they still live close to our inborn wish to be happy and free from suffering. One mother told me that using "we" is especially effective with young children ("May *we* be happy") because kids have a fluid sense of "I" and "mine." When helping older children become more self-compassionate, a useful question to ask is "What would your best friend say to you right now?" Once you've grounded yourself in the practice, use your creativity to explore the many ways to engage your children.

"Should I always think of my own needs first?"

We need to listen to one another to be happy in relationship. That means that we have to occasionally put our own needs aside and validate the experience of the other person. But as you read in the vignette about Suzanne and Michael in Chapter 1, we can't put our own needs aside to have a happy relationship unless the pain buried in our hearts is seen and heard, *at least by ourselves.*

Troy and Carlos had been living together for eight years and had a 4-year-old adopted son. Carlos came from a large, close-knit family that had loud, cantankerous arguments over the dinner table, whereas Troy's family of origin was quiet, often even sullen due to simmering resentments. Troy had a low tolerance for emotional outbursts because they had quickly become violent when he was a child. He was an introvert, and he calmed down in private. When Troy and Carlos had a disagreement over how to raise their son, Carlos demanded that Troy talk with him as Troy retreated into the bedroom to lie down. Carlos was an extravert, preferring to solve problems in the presence of others. As Troy pulled away, Carlos became agitated and spoke loudly; the pain of disconnection was too great for Carlos to bear, unfamiliar as it was from his family of origin. Carlos was left feeling wounded, and Troy felt threatened, leaving them no room to actually hear the hopes and dreams they each had for their child and how to incorporate them into how they raised him.

After 3 months of couple therapy, I asked this couple what they'd learned from treatment, if anything: "If there were only one thing to remember when you have an argument, what would that be?" Troy said, "Not to judge myself." (Troy felt like a "horrible person" when Carlos yelled at him.) Carlos said, "Open to unhappiness." Carlos had entered the relationship expecting that Troy's companionship would always feel good. He hadn't anticipated that Troy would pull away in an argument, making him feel lonely and abandoned. Troy and Carlos put their insights into practice. Carlos found that validating the unhappiness he felt as Troy retreated helped him "lay aside how it is for me, not even reluctantly, and then listen with openness and patience to figure out where Troy is coming from." That brought Troy out of his corner, and he reminded Carlos what a valuable companion he was.

Mindfulness and self-compassion can transform most of our personal relationships for the better—but only if we're willing to feel the inevitable pain that relationships entail. When we turn away from our distress, we abandon our loved ones as well as ourselves. But when we incline toward whatever is arising within us, we can be truly present and alive for one another.

"Will I ever overcome the urge to resist and avoid emotional pain?"

No. The instinct to push away pain is hardwired. A patient of mine once said, "The desire to not get upset is like hope—it springs eternal!" We will always have the potential for self-made suffering from trying to avoid emotional pain. Mindfulness and self-compassion practice can simply make those periods shorter and shorter.

Geoff was an exceptionally bright guy, a computer wizard, who felt anxious about many things: his kids, job, money, marriage, and physical health. Almost anything he paid attention to became a source of worry. In therapy, Geoff quickly understood the concept of "what you resist persists." He was the perfect client, diligently practicing formal meditation twice daily for 20 minutes and informally whenever he felt anxious during the day. After a month, when I asked if his efforts were paying off, Geoff said he wasn't sure. He still felt anxious despite all his hard work.

Geoff was in the "disillusionment" phase of treatment. He was practicing in order to be less anxious, to "comfort [anxiety] away," which is yet another form of resistance. Geoff was a workhorse and an intellectual—he understood how to work toward a goal, and it was taking him a little longer to get the *feeling* for self-compassion. With this insight, Geoff gradually shifted his emphasis from working *toward* self-compassion to just giving himself kindness when he felt bad. ("This hurts. May I live with ease.") He stopped seeing self-compassion as a "project" and started living in the present moment as an anxious guy who needs some loving.

Intellectual people initially believe that the *concept* of self-compassion is the thing itself, but conceptual understanding is only the first step. Resistance to discomfort is a subcortical process occurring at the gut level, and self-compassion becomes most effective when it operates at that level. But even when compassion is deep, resistance springs eternal. Practice is necessary as long as we reside in a human body.

"Does self-compassion ever become automatic?"

Yes, somewhat. Changes will occur in your life when you least expect them, such as when you lock your keys in your car or when you show up at an important meeting 1 hour late. You may be surprised to discover how understanding you've become ("I guess I've been overcommitted lately"), rather than self-critical ("You fool!").

I had client, Aiko, who had not heard of self-compassion before she began practicing it. Six months later, as Aiko was describing her daily schedule of crippling work deadlines, I wondered aloud whether she ever remembered to be compassionate with herself. Aiko replied that simply saying the word "compassion" made a tear trickle down her face and softened her body. Another client told me that the word "kindness" was all he needed to evoke the feeling. With sufficient practice, words like "kindness" or "compassion" can trigger a host of beneficial nonverbal responses—softening the body, allowing unpleasant feelings to pass through, and loving ourselves. At later stages, only a flash of awareness ("Ouch!") is enough to trigger a self-compassionate outcome.

"My problem is my own behavior! How do I change?"

All of us suffer from less-than-exemplary behaviors. Those actions often arise from our schemas—old habits of responding to threatening situations. Cesar, a middle-aged jazz musician, was a man with "mistrust" and "failure" schemas.

Cesar worked a daytime job in an office supply store and complained bitterly about the fact that his talents were not properly recognized and compensated for at this stage in his life. Whenever his boss at the store questioned something he did, such as how he talked to customers, Cesar responded sharply and angrily. Behavior like this had led to a succession of unsatisfactory jobs.

I had known Cesar for about 2 years when complaints about his supervisors started sounding repetitive. Cesar noticed the pattern as well. He confided in me that he had an anger problem, lamenting that "anger is like drinking poison and expecting someone else to die." Cesar saw how correcting the problem would have to be an inside job. I asked Cesar what criticism from his boss signified to him. "I won't be able to provide for my family," he said. "I'm all alone at work. I will never be able to make enough money to play music." Cesar broke it down even further: "I'm a failure."

We discussed kindness toward oneself as a way to transform anger at its roots. Cesar, an unusually creative person, decided to visualize a "wisdom figure with his arm around me" whenever he felt like a failure. In just a few weeks, Cesar found himself feeling less vulnerable at work, knowing he had a way of comforting himself when he felt attacked, and his angry retorts subsided.

Finding the soft feelings behind our hard feelings—in this case, the sense of failure behind angry words—gives us flexibility in how we behave in response to perceived threats. We're no longer condemned to act in habitual ways. We're not trying to directly change hard feelings—to drive them out—but rather to cultivate a *soft relationship to hard feelings* that gives them a chance to change on their own.

"Can't being soft open the door to getting taken advantage of? Is that really the best way to be?"

Many situations in life demand mental toughness. Some personalities, like the "floater" or people suffering from "weariness," may need to summon up inner strength to meet life's challenges. Their default option is to acquiesce, which can cause more suffering when they're caught in a bad situation. It's important to set limits on the behavior of others when they're hurting us.

Paula was a physical therapist, married for 4 years to a gentle, well-educated, handsome man, Kyle. His family of origin had a long history of alcoholism, and after a year of marriage, Kyle fell into the same trap. Paula felt sorry for him, and enjoyed his company when he was sober, but over time she found herself the family's sole financial provider and her partner less and less emotionally present. When she started flirting with a colleague over lunch, Paula decided that she needed to take steps to address her marital problem.

Kyle refused to acknowledge that he suffered from alcoholism, so Paula turned to Al-Anon for support. Over the following 3 years Paula felt alternately sorry for Kyle and enraged at his emotional and financial abandonment of her and their two kids and his unwillingness to stop drinking. Paula's struggle was validated at Al-Anon meetings, which gave her the courage to seek legal advice about divorce. Upon getting this news, Kyle still refused to admit he had a problem, blaming Paula and his unhappy marriage for his drinking. Paula always considered divorce to be a last resort, and she felt terrible about it, as if God would be disappointed with her. She was caught up in shame and blame. Paula gradually opened up to the anguish of returning every evening from work to her husband watching TV with a martini. "I deserve to be happy," Paula heard herself saying. "I too need moments of leisure. I don't deserve to be lonely, angry, and miserable all the time." Paula left her husband.

When we pay attention to our inner experience and accept how we *truly* feel—unhappy, lacking direction, empty, ashamed, despairing—we're likely to discover a huge reservoir of strength and determination. Like a mother defending her young, internal softness often leads to external toughness. The foundation for setting limits on others is knowing our *own* limits.

"If it's my current attitude toward pain and suffering that's so crucial for emotional healing, does that mean I should just leave my past behind?"

This question echoes many discussions I've had with psychotherapists who were trained to explore their patients' early childhood experiences. It's indeed important to understand how our past has shaped us. Our core emotional habits are meaningful objects for mindful self-compassion (see self-schemas in Chapter 4) and knowing the details of our lives help us to accept them more fully.

Remember Michelle, the young woman described in Chapter 1 who couldn't control her blushing? Michelle had always been a highly sensitive person, more so than her three brothers. Her father was quite stern and didn't mince words when he was upset with the kids. Michelle was also a beautiful child who received a lot of attention for her appearance, but schoolwork didn't come easily to her. She dreaded each September when school began, especially after a carefree summer. Michelle applied herself with diligence to her schoolwork and eventually succeeded in graduating from a good university.

Deep inside, however, Michelle always felt like an imposter. She had vastly exceeded the achievements of her parents, which she believed was due to hard work rather than her intelligence or competence, and she had internalized the critical messages of her father. When Michelle went on job interviews, she was sure her inadequacies would be exposed, especially if the interviewer was a male.

Michelle had a brief infatuation with therapy after she discovered that acceptance-based strategies stopped her blushing. But infatuation quickly led to disillusionment, which lingered for many months. It just wasn't enough to "accept" that she blushed—something deeper had to be addressed. Ironically, Michelle had a breakthrough when she became depressed during the fall season. She couldn't understand why she was feeling that way until she connected it with school resuming and how terrible she always felt at that time of year. "My father always told me that I was not as smart as my brothers. I could never prove him otherwise. It felt awful."

With that insight, Michelle started feeling the pain left deep in her heart. To accept blushing meant being a total failure—unlovable. Michelle started to grieve those many years of academic struggle and self-doubt, allowing herself just to feel sad about it. Somehow she started to feel more human and in her body. Michelle became more patient with the therapy process as well, knowing how deeply her feelings ran. She gave herself 3 years to learn to be more self-accepting in response to blushing. To assist the process, Michelle visualized Jesus tapping her on the shoulder whenever she felt bad. When she started to blush, she added, "May I love myself just as I am." I recently called Michelle, 1 year after we last met, to get permission to write her story. She told me she hardly ever thinks of blushing anymore.

Self-compassion has the "gleam of the particulars," as poet Naomi Shihab Nye might say. The details of our lives are necessary to contact the deeper meaning of our daily experience. In the case of Michelle, she couldn't fully connect with her emotional pain—get a visceral sense of it—until she understood its origin and the long trajectory it took in her life. Then she had a deep and authentic experience to address with self-compassion. Self-compassion is not a strategy for bypassing our personal issues—it helps us to have a full life *within* them.

"Self-compassion has done a lot for me, but is it an emotional cure-all?"

There's always an element of self-compassion—caring for ourselves and allowing ourselves to be happy—when life is flowing smoothly. We should be cautious, however, about pushing self-compassion on ourselves in all situations. Sometimes we need to turn away from our pain to make it manageable, sometimes we should take medication, and other times we should do nothing at all. Self-compassion is not a universal panacea.

There are also occasions when we need to take a tough attitude toward our emotions. That doesn't mean denying them, but rather it means that certain circumstances—abuse, war, working as a paramedic—require that we focus exclusively on the task at hand until we can process our feelings later on. The challenges in our lives are too diverse to respond to self-compassion alone, but, in combination with other tools at our disposal, self-compassion can make life a whole lot easier. Ultimately, what makes our lives happier in the long run is the compassionate thing to do.

It may sound strange, but I generally try to avoid the term "self-compassion" while counseling others because it creates a standard against which we all inevitably fail. Self-compassion isn't a "thing" that we either *have* or *don't have*. Instead, as a practitioner and as a therapist, I try to remain open to emotional pain and breathe kindness into it, one moment after the next.

MEASURING YOUR PROGRESS

Self-compassion is a long-term adventure. You'll recognize changes in yourself almost immediately, but an underlying shift in attitude is a slow, incremental process. It's best to take the long view—give yourself a lifetime to practice, but make sure you notice progress along the way. *Haba na haba, hujaza kibaba* (Swahili for "Little by little fills the pot"). Or, as my good friend and meditation teacher Trudy Goodman said, "Self-compassion is never fixed, never having arrived."

Self-Compassion Scale

If you completed the Self-Compassion Scale when you read about it in Chapter 4, you can retest yourself now to see how you're doing. See if your scores on self-kindness, common humanity, and mindfulness go up, and if your scores on self-judgment, isolation, and overidentification go down.

Self-Compassion Journal

One month is a sufficient period of time to discover the transformative power of self-compassion. Within 2 months, you're likely to go through both the infatuation and the disillusionment phases. I often recommend to beginning practitioners that they keep a journal for at least *3 months* to explore the vicissitudes of practice. Journaling is an opportunity to monitor habit change, to troubleshoot, and, most important, to notice new ways you might be responding to problems in your life. The simple act of writing also reinforces your commitment.

Make your journal simple and easy to use. You can keep an open document in your computer, e-mail a daily entry to yourself, or just jot down notes on a pad kept in your purse or pocket. Record the subtle changes, such as the kindly words that might appear unexpectedly in your mind. If you're not the writing type, make a mental note of changes or mention them to others who might be interested in your progress. A Self-Compassion Journal might look like this:

Day 12

Slept poorly last night and feeling edgy. Sitting meditation for 20 minutes after coffee. Meditated to feel better, which didn't work at all. When I just let myself feel crummy and say the phrases, I felt better. I continued the phrases on way to work, but then forgot the whole day. Super busy. Will try again before I go to sleep.

Day 13

Slept better last night, maybe because of the phrases? No time to meditate today. Consciously enjoyed the warm water in my shower, though. That was different. Since I didn't meditate, I promised myself to say the phrases more often during the day. When my phone rang, I noticed on caller ID that it was the day care center. I said "safe, safe, safe" and then picked up the phone. A first! There was no problem, but I felt better anyway.

<u>Day 14</u>

Sat for 10 min this morning. It helped to envision that before I got out of bed. I'd prefer 20 min. Didn't get past the breath part in 10 min. Helps to think beforehand that I'm sitting just to be with myself before a busy day and let everything be just as it is. It's the only time of the day like that. Usually I'm trying to accomplish something.

The old car rattle started again on the way home. %$#@&*! I mean, METTA!

<u>Day 15</u>

Woke up saying, "Don't be afraid." Haven't got a clue where that came from. I'm hardcore! Mornings are getting a little less crazy, maybe because I'm going to bed earlier. It's still a pain trying to get Josh out the door. Maybe I'll sing the metta phrases to him. It couldn't hurt Josh to grow up knowing this stuff.

Keeping a journal is itself a contemplative practice and a self-compassion exercise. You're honoring the preciousness of your own experience, even if it's odd, funky, or confusing.

If you're having trouble getting started with journaling, try picking a specific problem, such as resentment toward a lazy colleague who gets all the credit at work, and document what you're doing and how it's going. Perhaps you started saying "May I love myself just as I am." How is it going? Also, note when you *forget* to practice—the slippery slope back to old habits—and brainstorm how to support yourself.

Avoid the trap of evaluating your progress *while* you're meditating. You may or may not have a positive state of mind and still be making progress. While practicing, stick to the practice itself.

That means that if you feel bad, deliver kindness to yourself. Or anchor your attention in your breath, or sit back and watch the inner drama in a generous, openhearted way. Stay engaged in the present moment, and don't judge how it worked until you're done.

You *can* measure your progress by how you feel in your daily life. Are you feeling happier, more confident, less stressed? More important, are you responding with more and more good will toward yourself when things go wrong? When you banged your knee on the coffee table, did you say, "Ouch! That hurts! God love you!" or did you blurt out, "You clumsy jerk!" Are you trading self-criticism, self-isolation, and self-absorption for self-kindness, a sense of your humanness, and the ability to let go? If so, make a note.

BEGINNING ANEW

The path to happiness and well-being never ends. Just when we think we've arrived, a new challenge presents itself and we begin again. This book was written to help dissolve the illusion that we can better ourselves to the point where emotional pain is a thing of

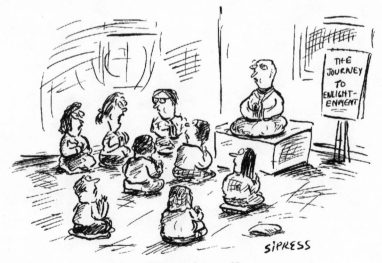

"Are we there yet?"

the past. A more fruitful path is to cultivate uncommon kindness—kindness toward ourselves—as long as we live and breathe. In the words of meditation teacher Pema Chödrön: "... we can still be crazy after all these years. We can still be angry after all these years. We can still be timid or jealous or full of feelings of unworthiness. The point is ... not to try to throw ourselves away and become something better. It's about befriending who we are already."

It could make all the difference in your life.

APPENDIX A

emotion words

The following list of emotion words was compiled from an online search by computer linguist Steven DeRose. It attests to the subtlety and diversity of human emotional experience. The list can be used to find a label for almost any emotion you're likely to have in daily life.

This list, as well as the author's sources, can also be found at *www.derose.net/steve/resources/emotionwords/ewords.html.*

Reprinted by permission of Steven J. DeRose.

PAIN/PLEASURE

Angry

acrimonious, angry, annoyed, appalled, bitter, boiling, cross, devastated, disgusted, enraged, frustrated, fuming, furious, hostile, in a huff, in a stew, incensed, indignant, inflamed, infuriated, irate, irritated, livid, mad, offended, outraged, piqued, provoked, rageful, resentful, sullen, up in arms, virulent, worked up, wrathful, wrought up

Sad

aching, afflicted, agonized, anguished, bereaved, blue, cheerless, clouded, crestfallen, crushed, dark, dejected, depressed, despairing, despondent, disconsolate, discontented, discouraged, disheartened, dismal, displeased, distressed, dolorous, down, downcast, downhearted, dreadful, dreary, dull, embarrassed, flat, frowning, funereal, gloomy, glum, griefstricken, grieved, guilt, hapless, heartbroken, heavyhearted, humiliated, hurt, ill at ease, in despair, in pain, in the dumps, injured, joyless, lonely, low-spirited, low, lugubrious, melancholy, moody, moping, mournful, offended, oppressed, out of sorts, pathetic, piteous, regretful, remorse, rueful, shamed, shocked, somber, sorrowful, spiritless, suffering, sulky, sullen, tortured, tragic, unhappy, woebegone, woeful, worried

Happy

airy, amused, animated, beatific, blissful, blithe, bright, brisk, buoyant, cheerful, cheery, comfortable, contented, convivial, debonair, ecstatic, elated, enthusiastic, excited, exhilarated, exultant, festive, free and easy, frisky, genial, glad, gleeful, great, high-spirited, hilarious, humorous, important, inspired, jaunty, jocular, jolly, jovial, joyful, joyous, jubilant, laughing, lighthearted, lively, lucky, merry, mirthful, overjoyed, peaceful, playful, pleased, proud, rapturous, satisfied, saucy, self-satisfied, serene, sparkling, spirited, sprightly, sunny, terrific, thankful, tranquil, transported, vivacious

Ecstatic

delighted, fabulous, fantastic, overjoyed

POWER/CONTROL/RESPONSIBILITY

Irresistible

aggressive, exuberant, immortal, indestructible, invincible, invulnerable, powerful, unstoppable

Powerless

bashful, blocked, defeated, discouraged, disorganized, exhausted, hopeless, irresponsible, overwhelmed, thwarted, worn down, worn out

Out of Control

careless, impotent, obligated, obliterated, powerless, reckless, vulnerable, weak

Apathetic

complacent, full of ennui, immobilized, lazy, lethargic, numb, passive, quiescent, unconcerned, unmotivated

Adequate

capable, competent, composed, confident, encouraged, excited, in control, organized, responsible

ATTACHMENT

Alone

cut off, excluded, forsaken, isolated, left out, rejected, shut out, detached, lonely, lonesome, misunderstood

Independent

arrogant, autonomous, cocky, strong, macho

Attached

affectionate, belonging, captivated, cherished, compassionate, connected, empathetic, included, liked, loved, loving, understood

Codependent

addicted, insecure, needy, sympathetic

Hated

abandoned, chastised, criticized, deserted, discarded, forsaken, ignored, left out, let down, overlooked, rejected, replaced, unapproved of, unlovable, unloved

Loved

accepted, adored, adorable, approved of, desirable, entrusted, loved, validated, valued, welcomed

SOCIAL STANDING

Belittled

chagrined, diminished, discredited, disgraced, insignificant, underestimated, unsupported

Embarrassed

ashamed, awkward, disparaged, guilty

Average

common, ordinary

Esteemed

admired, appreciated, respected, revered, significant, supported, valued, worshiped

JUSTICE

Cheated

disparaged, victimized

Singled Out

affronted, categorized, guilty, judged, labeled, rated, stereotyped

Justified

absolved, acquitted, appeased, redeemed, satisfied, vindicated

Entitled

exempt, favored, immune, privileged

FREEDOM

Trapped

imprisoned, optionless

Burdened

obligated, pressured, put upon, thwarted

Free

autonomous, independent, released, unshackled

DIRECTION/FOCUS

Derailed

disjointed, disoriented, torn

Lost

baffled, bewildered, confused, unfocused

Focused

committed, complacent, determined, in the zone

Obsessed

compelled, consumed

DESIRE/INTEREST

Demoralized

disappointed, discouraged, disheartened, disillusioned, disinclined, repulsed, stifled, thwarted

Bored

ambivalent, apathetic, complacent, full of ennui, indifferent, lackadaisical, unmotivated

Attracted

absorbed, affected, agog, full of anticipation, anxious, attracted, avid, challenged, concerned, confident, craving, curious, dedicated, desirous, eager, earnest, enchanted, engrossed, enthusiastic, excited, fascinated, fervent, fervid, hopeful, inquisitive, inspiring, intent, interested, intrigued, keen, motivated, needed, nosey, snoopy, zealous

Lustful

addicted, ardent, aroused, horny, hot and bothered, infatuated, lustful, needy, passionate, turned on, yearning

SAFETY/SECURITY

Fearful

afraid, aghast, alarmed, anxious, appalled, apprehensive, awed, cautious, chicken, cowardly, defenseless, diffident, dismayed, doubtful, exposed, fainthearted, fearful, fidgety, frightened, hesitant, horrified, hysterical, in fear, insecure, irresolute, menaced, misgiving, nervous, panicked, petrified, phobic, quaking, restful, scared, shaky, shocked, suspicious, terrified, terrorized, timid, timorous, trembling, tremulous, upset, worried, yellow

Anxious

apprehensive, cautious, concerned, distrustful, doubtful, dubious, full of misgiving, hesitant, indecisive, pensive, perplexed, questioning, skeptical, suspicious, tense, unbelieving, uncertain, uncomfortable, wavering

Fearless

audacious, bold, brave, certain, confident, courageous, daring, dauntless, determined, encouraged, enterprising, gallant, hardy, heroic, reassured, resolute, secure, self-reliant, spirited, stout-hearted

Safe

at ease, calm, comfortable, composed, peaceful, secure

Surprise

astonished, bewildered, confused, shocked, startled, surprised

MISCELLANEOUS

active, afraid, agitated, animosity, antagonistic, artificial, astounded, aware

bad, balanced, beautiful, blurry

childish, clear, clever, competitive, complexity, conciliated, conspicuous, constrained, contemptuous, courteous, cruel, cynical

deceitful, decisive, defiant, dependent, desperate, destructive, different, dim, disqualified, disregarded, dissatisfied, distracted, disturbed, divided, drained, droopy, dumb earthy, embittered, empty, energetic, enlightened, envious, evil, exasperated

failure, fatigued, firm, flustered, fond, foolish, forgiving, fortunate, frank, frantic, friendly, frozen, fulfilled, full, futile

generous, giddy, good, grateful, greedy, gullible

harried, hasty, haughty, helpful, helpless, homesick, honored, horrible

imposed upon, impressed, inadequate, incapable, incompetent, inconsiderate, ineffective, inferior, intense, intimidated, intricate, involved

jealous, jumpy

kind

lenient, longing, lovable

mature, mean, meditative, methodical, miserable, misery, mocked, murderous

natural, naughty, nice

obnoxious, odd, optimistic, out of place

pained, patient, perturbed, pessimistic, pitied, pleasant, posing, possessive, pretty, pushy, put down, puzzled

relaxed, relieved, respected, responsive, restless, restrained, revengeful, rewarded, ridiculous, right, routine

skeptical, scornful, self-confident, self-doubt, servile, sharp, shy, sick, silly, sincerity, sleepy, slumber, smart, sneaky, solemn, spiteful, stable, stingy, strange, stressed, stubborn, stunned, stupid, successful, suicidal, superior, sure talkative, tempted, tenacious, tender, tentative, terrible, tired, tolerant, troubled, trusted

ugly, unaware, undecided, undeserving, undesirable, uneasy, unequaled, unfair, unfulfilled, unified, unmatched, unsettled, unsupported, unstable, unsure, unwanted, unworthy, uptight, useless

vehement, vigilant, vile, violent, vitriolic

weary, whimsical, wicked, wiped out, wonderful, worthless, worthy

APPENDIX B

additional self-compassion exercises

A self-compassion exercise is any practice that enhances good will toward ourselves when we suffer. Loving-kindness (*metta*) meditation has been emphasized in this book because it changes the inner dialogue that has a large impact on how we feel. Other pathways to self-compassion were mentioned in Chapter 5, and more can be found in the books and audio materials listed in Appendix C. The additional practices described below were selected due to their unique nature or broad appeal.

GIVING AND TAKING MEDITATION (*TONGLEN*)

This unusual meditation uses the ordinary process of breathing, coordinating it with the mental practice of inhaling suffering and exhaling ease and well-being. "*Inhaling* suffering?" you say. "Shouldn't it be the reverse, inhaling ease and *exhaling* suffering? Am I not just building up suffering inside?" The beauty of this meditation is that with every breath it reverses our instinctive tendency to avoid or resist negative experience. By intentionally drawing pain inside, we undermine the mental habit of resistance that creates and perpetuates suffering. That's a compassionate thing to do.

Giving and taking meditation is attributed to the Buddhist teacher Atisha Dipankara Shrijnana, who lived in India in the 10th century CE. *Tong* means "giving" in the Tibetan language and *len* means "taking." (It's actually practiced *len-tong,* taking and giving.) The purpose of this mind-training technique is to develop compassion toward all beings, including oneself. The foremost Western proponent of giving and taking meditation is Pema Chödrön, an American nun in the Tibetan Buddhist tradition. Her books listed in Appendix C, especially *Tonglen,* offer a wealth of insight into the practice. The following series of meditation instructions are adapted from Pema Chödrön's instructions and specifically emphasize self-compassion. They can be practiced as a sitting meditation for 10–20 minutes, or informally whenever you feel the need.

- Sit quietly for a few moments.

- Take a few conscious breaths, breathing in and out through all the pores of your body. *Feel* your breath as you inhale and as you exhale. You might want to imagine your body as a balloon that is being inflated with every in-breath. Do this until your attention is anchored in your breathing.

- Open yourself to *physical* sensation in your body and locate any discomfort. If you have any, where is it located? Your stomach, chest, neck, or head?

- Now focus on your heart area and see if you're carrying any *emotional* distress. If so, what's its *texture*? Does it feel "thick," "turbulent," "hard," "rough," or "heavy"? How does it *look* in your mind's eye? Does it appear "dark," "gray," or "murky"? Try to get a sense of the discomfort so you can clearly identify it. Give it a name, if you wish, such as "pain," "discouraged," or "worried."

- Link your discomfort to your breath. With every in-breath, draw *in* your distress. Take a rich, full breath. Inhale the discomfort from wherever it's located in your body.

- Imagine that your discomfort is being transformed in the gap between your in- and out-breaths, perhaps by light in the center of your being or simply on its own.

- Breathe out spaciousness and relief to yourself and others. Breathe from your center through your own body, suffusing it with well-being, and into the world.

- Let your out-breath be the opposite of your in-breath. If you are breathing in darkness, send out light. If you're inhaling tightness, exhale softness. If you're breathing in roughness, send out smoothness. Practice in a way that you can feel the difference. If you're visualizing your body as an empty balloon, let the air out, releasing clean, pure air to all beings. You can send out ease and well-being to specific needy persons or to the world in general.

- Feel free to take more than one breath to inhale suffering or to exhale well-being, until you get the hang of it. Then let your breath gradually settle into a natural, easy rhythm, breathing *in* your distress and breathing *out* kindness and well-being.

- Close your meditation by sitting quietly, allowing your entire internal experience to be just as it is.

Tonglen meditation depends on our ability to release sticky feelings—to draw them in and freely let them go. That's why Pema Chödrön's instructions suggest we breathe through all the pores of the skin or visualize our bodies like an empty balloon—there's less to stick to. That's also the reason we just sit quietly and let go of all effort before and after tonglen practice.

Tonglen meditation contains many of the underlying healing mechanisms we talked about earlier in this book. It uses the calming power of focused attention on the breath, it anchors the ruminative mind in the body, it reverses the tendency to avoid or resist emotional pain, it encourages balanced awareness of pain, it nourishes good will, and it generates a greater sense of connection with others.

My 34-year-old niece helped me recognize the healing aspect of *connection* in tonglen practice.

My niece is the mother of two beautiful daughters, a 2- and a 4-year-old. Her 4-year-old was going through a difficult phase at a family gathering, crying and fussing a lot. She confided in me how painful it was to hear her daughter cry and was at a loss for how to help her daughter, or herself, feel better. As a busy mother, she had no time to meditate and barely enough time to breathe. I wondered whether tonglen meditation might help and taught it to her in just a few minutes.

At breakfast the following morning, my niece told me the practice worked wonders—it helped her stay calm even though her daughter continued to be distraught. When I asked how that worked, she explained that she inhaled her distress and frustration and exhaled love to her daughter. The practice allowed her to "stay close to [my daughter] without losing myself." By wanting the crying to stop, my niece was unconsciously distancing herself from her daughter and suffered the pain of a crying child *plus* the pain of disconnection. Tonglen meditation helped her get her daughter back.

I know another woman, Celine, who uses tonglen to alleviate her distress when she sees signs of aging—new wrinkles, sagging jowls—in the mirror in the morning. Celine inhales the anxiety of the woman in the mirror, and as she exhales, Celine says, "Darling, you're just getting older. So is everyone else. Everyone is growing old together."

Tonglen can be practiced when we're distressed in any way. Workhorse personalities seem to like tonglen because, with a little practice, it slips effortlessly into a busy day. Extraverts may enjoy the connection aspect and that it's slightly less psychological than metta meditation—more rooted in the bodily process of breathing. Generally speaking, people who enjoy their bodies may take easily to tonglen. Tonglen practitioners with experience in metta practice can try reciting the metta phrases along with each tonglen out-breath, sending loving-kindness to all. Find what works for you.

Modifications to Giving and Taking Meditation

Opening to emotional pain can be overwhelming at times no matter what method we use. If that happens during tonglen practice, there are a few modifications that I've found useful. For example, if you're *very* overwhelmed, try this:

- Sit quietly for a few moments.

- Take a few breaths through all the pores of your body and also breathe out through all the pores of your body.

- Think of a few people who love you and place them in a circle around you. Locate them as close to or as far away from you as you like. Visualize them patiently sitting, just for you, with love and care in their hearts. You can also visualize your favorite pets or see yourself in a natural setting, surrounded by beauty.

- Place your hand on your heart.

- Continue consciously breathing. As you inhale, breathe in their love. As you exhale, return the love. Get a sense of inhaling warmth and kindness and exhaling gratitude and love.

- Breathe in and out as long as you wish, feeling the energy of loving-kindness radiating toward you and from you as you breathe.

- Gently open your eyes.

This adaptation steers you *away* from suffering and is suitable when you're deeply upset. When you're less upset—perhaps merely "disturbed"—you can open yourself to a little more suffering, but be sure you still give loving-kindness to yourself as well. The following spectrum of tonglen modifications correspond to how distressed you may be when you practice:

- *Overwhelmed?*   Take loving-kindness from those who love you. Give loving-kindness to those who love you.

- *Disturbed?*   Take in your own suffering. Give loving-kindness to *yourself.*

- *Distressed?*   Take in your own suffering. Give loving-kindness to *yourself and others.*

- *Dissatisfied?*   Take in your suffering *and the suffering of others.* Give loving-kindness to *others.*

- *Content?*   Take in others' suffering. Give others loving-kindness.

You may notice that the very first set of tonglen instructions given above—taking your *own* suffering and giving loving-kindness to *yourself and others*—is practiced in the middle range of discomfort ("distressed"). If you're feeling better than that—only "dissatisfied"—try connecting your pain to the pain of millions of others on the planet who might be feeling exactly the same way in the present moment. For example, if you have a stomachache, think of all the people who have stomachaches. Draw that common pain into your body with the in-breath, transmute it, and breathe out ease and well-being to all. You might get relief from the feeling of not being so alone in your struggle.

If you're feeling "content," try taking on the suffering of others and giving out love to others. That is traditional tonglen practice, designed for liberation from the prison of our own individuality. When the Dalai Lama was asked how he meditates, especially to cultivate forgiveness, he responded:

> I use meditation technique called giving and taking . . . I make visualization: send my positive emotions like happiness, affection to others. Then another visualization. I visualize receiving their sufferings, their negative emotions. I do this every day. I pay special attention to the Chinese—especially those doing terrible things to the Tibetans. So, as I meditate, I breathe in all their poisons—hatred, fear, cruelty. Then I breathe out. And I let all the good things come out, things like compassion, forgiveness. I take inside my body all these bad things. Then I replace poisons with fresh air. Giving and taking. I take care not to blame—I don't blame the Chinese and I don't blame myself. This meditation is very effective, useful to reduce hatred, useful to cultivate forgiveness.

Most of us don't have the compassion of the Dalai Lama, or his peace of mind, so we are advised to practice with the other modifications as well.

CENTERING MEDITATION

Centering meditation is a technique for discovering a compassionate word or phrase that applies particularly to you and your current situation. Beginning practitioners of loving-kindness meditation can use centering meditation to discover their own personalized metta phrases.

Centering meditation comes from a 14th-century anonymously written book called *The Cloud of Unknowing,* which was discovered in the attic of a Trappist monastery in Spencer, Massachusetts. Centering became popular in 1982 through Father Basil Pennington's *Centering Prayer: Renewing an Ancient Christian Prayer Form.* The meditation is designed to open our hearts and minds to inner guidance that is beyond our usual habits of thought. The following meditation is a secularized version of that technique. Like many other meditations, the prescribed length of time is about 20 minutes, once or twice a day.

- Sit comfortably, close your eyes, and take a few deep, relaxing breaths.

- Notice your posture—sitting, not lying down, not standing—and feel any sensations in your body. If you have any physical discomfort, gently touch it with your awareness. If you have emotional distress, notice it and let it be there.

- Now bring attention to your *breathing,* wherever you feel it most strongly. Nostrils? Chest? Belly? When your mind wanders, gently return to the sensation of breathing. As you breathe, let your awareness move deeply into the experience of breathing. Do this for 5–10 minutes.

- The breath comes seemingly out of nowhere—it's actually breathing *you,* keeping you healthy even when you're fast asleep. Go deeply into the breath, to the *source* of the breath. Let your awareness drop into the deep, empty space from which breathing emerges, from which the faintest movement originates. This place, beyond thoughts and words, is a field of great peace and freedom.

- Just continue to breathe and open your awareness to the source of your breath. As you do so, listen for any words that may bubble up. Open yourself up to a word or a phrase that might be *just what you need to hear right now.* If a word or phrase were to appear from the bottom of your heart, what would it be?

- Take a few minutes to do this. Breathe, relax, and open yourself to words that might bubble up from deep inside. If no words arise, just stay with your breath. If a *few* words arise, roll them over in your mind and select one that's perfect for you at this time in your life. Some possibilities might be "love," "let it be," "I love you," "yes," "trust," "peace" or "mercy."

- When you have a word or phrase, allow yourself to savor it, rolling it over and over in your mind. If you notice that your mind has wandered, bring it ever so gently back to the word or words.

- After a while, let go of what you're doing and simply be with your inner experience, letting yourself be just as you are.

- Slowly open your eyes.

It can be a stirring experience to hear encouraging words coming from the depths of one's being, such as "I love you," "Let go and let God," or "Have courage." An intellectual client of mine, an electrical engineer with attention-deficit/hyperactivity disorder (ADHD), heard "Don't be afraid." The words stirred him to tears, unsure why they came up since they seemed unrelated to his usual way of thinking. Then he heard "Focus!," a familiar admonition from his childhood. He wisely selected "Don't be afraid" as his centering phrase. Another client with ADHD heard the word "dynamo" while he did the centering meditation, and he felt it energized him when his mind wandered off task.

Centering meditation is essentially mantra meditation with a twist: the mantra is self-generated. A mantra is commonly used in meditation to disentangle us from meaningless thinking and calm the mind through one-pointed attention. Depending on the religious tradition, sometimes the *meaning* of the mantra is important, sometimes it's the *sound,* sometimes it's *writing* the mantra that matters, and often a mantra is just a meaningless, yet helpful, object of attention.

The sound of the body exhaling, "Ahhhhhhh, ahhhhhhh, ahhhh-hhh," is a mantra, and can be comforting when you feel under stress. Repeating a name of God, particularly if you feel loved by God, can be a compelling way to use a mantra to cultivate self-compassion. A name of God (Jesus, Ram) may come to mind during centering meditation or can be brought in from your religious tradition.

Centering meditation can also have a surprisingly beneficial effect on people who are likely to feel alone or unloved, such as outsiders, survivors, or perfectionists. They feel connected to a deeper, more loving part of themselves. The butterfly and floater personalities may also benefit from centering meditation by learning to trust inner guidance.

LIGHT MEDITATION

"The light of love." "The clear light of awareness." "Shed some light on the matter." Light is a universal symbol for virtuous qualities such as love, truth, and wisdom. When we visualize light within ourselves, we affirm our good qualities.

The following meditation may be familiar to people from different meditative traditions and has been modified here for self-compassion. Readers who are good at visualization, those who prefer nonverbal meditation, or intellectuals who like to work with abstract images are likely to enjoy light meditation.

A number of different mental tasks are involved in light meditation, so give yourself sufficient time, perhaps 15–20 minutes, to practice in a relaxed, unhurried manner. The point is to savor inner warmth, not to finish quickly.

- Light a candle and place it before you. Sit comfortably with a reasonably straight back and take a few deep, relaxing breaths. Gaze at the candle for a minute as it quietly emanates light in all directions. Gently close your eyes.

- Visualize the candlelight in the heart region of your body, as an unwavering flame or an orb of light. Let it shine in all directions just like a candle.

- Continue to rest your attention in your heart area. Feel the soft glow of candlelight in your heart. If you wish, you can open and close your eyes a few times, seeing the flame before you and then visualizing the flame in your heart.

- When your mind wanders, bring it ever so gently back to the light in your heart.

- Now begin to slowly move the light to different parts of your body. If you are feeling discomfort in any part of your body, let the light linger there awhile longer before moving onward.

  First bring it to your head. Let the light illuminate your brain.

  Then, going back down through your heart region, bring it through your arms to your hands, one arm after another. Take all the time you need.

  Again starting at your heart, now bring the light down your trunk and legs to your feet—one leg and then the next.

  Then bring the light back to your heart. If you have any emotional pain, allow the discomfort to be there while you suffuse your heart with light.

- Now let the light expand outside yourself, to include others in your room or house, your country, and the entire world. In your mind's eye, visualize yourself and your entire surroundings suffused with warm, radiant light.

- Slowly open your eyes when you're ready.

You can move the light anywhere you wish. If you want to keep it to yourself, feel free to do so. Personalities like caregivers and extraverts may want to share the light with everyone, and introverts may feel more comfortable nestled within themselves. After a few weeks of practice, you probably won't need to use a candle anymore, nor will you need to scan the body with light—you'll be able to suffuse your body with light at a moment's notice.

Don't try to be too literal about light meditation, or any visualization meditation. You don't have to actually "see" the candle in your mind's eye as you saw it outside—just let there be a sense of illumination in your heart region. When you close your eyes, you'll see light patterns on your eyelids. This is possible because you're a conscious being and your nerve cells contain energy. Every cell of your body contains energy. Let yourself be aware of the energy—pulsation, light, vitality—in your chest cavity.

Remember that the light is not intended to drive away negative feelings or qualities. It dispels darkness by its very nature, not by "trying." The warmth of light is like a heating pad that can be applied to a painful muscle. Simply apply the treatment when and where it's needed and see what happens.

MUSIC MEDITATION

Music can be a meditation when we're absorbed in it. Meditation, in the broadest sense, is a method of regulating attention and awareness for a particular purpose. Sometimes music is relaxing, sometimes it's stimulating, and often it moves us wordlessly into states of heightened perception and emotional awareness. When we use music to evoke good will toward ourselves, by focusing our attention and allowing loving feelings to arise, it becomes a self-compassion meditation.

Music can provide comfort in the midst of suffering. Pachelbel's "Canon" helped a dear friend who was dying of cancer accept her illness. When I play the song "I Will Always Love You" (Whitney Houston) in a workshop, it always moves a few people to tears. The key when listening to music is to *allow* yourself to be moved.

Music is a universal language—it can be enjoyed by all the personality types—but it's also highly subjective. Make your own "self-compassion play list." You can reinterpret some familiar love songs to bring love to yourself such as "I Will Always Love You" or "Stand by Me." Others, like Anna Nalick's "Just Breathe" or "All the Good in This Life" by Garbage, are explicitly self-compassionate. Devotional music, like Josh Groban's "You Raise Me Up," can awaken a deep sense of love, softening how we look at both the world and ourselves.

Here's a random selection of music to get you started:

"Dear Lord"/John Coltrane Quartet

"Close to You"/The Carpenters

Finale, Symphony No. 9: "Ode to Joy"/Ludwig van Beethoven

"When I'm Sixty-Four"/The Beatles

"You Are the Sunshine of My Life"/Stevie Wonder

"Our Love Is Here to Stay"/Ella Fitzgerald

"Angel"/Jimi Hendrix

"Jesu, Joy of Man's Desiring"/Johann Sebastian Bach

"Dedicated to the One I Love"/The Mamas and the Papas

Piano Sonata, Op. 109: first movement/Ludwig van Beethoven

Finale, Suite from *The Firebird*/Igor Stravinsky

"Reach Out, I'll Be There"/Four Tops

Traumerei, Op. 15, #7/Robert Schumann

"If You Love Somebody, Set Them Free"/Sting

"I Hear a Symphony"/The Supremes

Fantasie in C, third movement/Robert Schumann

"Everybody Is a Star"/Sly and the Family Stone

"Thank You (Falletinme Be Mice Elf Agin)"/Sly and the Family Stone

Sonata No. 2: first movement, Andante/Alexander Scriabin

"Lean on Me"/Ben E. King

"Acknowledgement," from *A Love Supreme*/John Coltrane Quartet

"Til the Morning Comes"/Grateful Dead

Being in Dreaming/Michael Hewett

"Welcome"/John Coltrane Quartet

A Meeting by the River/Ry Cooder and V. M. Bhatt

NATURE MEDITATION

As Georgia O'Keeffe said, "A flower touches everyone's heart." Wilderness areas and national parks have become the pilgrimage centers of the secular world, where we go for refuge, connection, and healing. When we walk in nature, we inevitably imagine ourselves as big as the sky, as solid as a tree, or as deep as a lake. If you sit long enough in the woods, listening quietly, the inhabitants of the forest will come out to be with you. Nature meditation may be especially healing to the survivor and the outsider. It offers a special way of practicing self-compassion when contact with people is, or has been, difficult.

The natural world is a great teacher. Nature continuously reveals birth and death, heat and cold, wet and dry, light and dark—the truth of impermanence. It can also be cruel, showing the universality of suffering. Nature is way too grand and beautiful to possess or control. Only by letting go and allowing ourselves to be vulnerable and moved by it can we share in nature's wealth. That's meditation.

My wife and I have a cabin in the Maine woods without electricity or running water. I go there, as John Burroughs wrote, "to be soothed and healed, and to have my senses put in tune once more." My wife doesn't have a formal meditation practice, but when she steps into the woods, her eyes sparkle with joy. She feels a sense of aliveness and interconnection that escapes most of us living in the concrete jungle.

For a compassionate guide to nature meditation, read *Awake in the Wild: Mindfulness in Nature as a Path in Self-Discovery* by Mark Coleman. This book contains instructions for meditating in nature and will make an excellent companion on your next walk in the woods.

MAKING A VOW

The subtext of this book is "intention, intention, intention," and making a vow can strengthen our core intentions. A vow is generally considered a solemn promise, but it's better to think of it as something gentle and light. It's a touchstone to which we return again and again, for the joy of it, as we might return to the breath in meditation. A vow turns life into meditation.

The loving-kindness phrases can double as a vow. For example, when I wake up in the morning, I try to remember the phrases:

> *May all beings be safe and free from harm.*
> *May all beings be peaceful and happy.*
> *May all beings be healthy and strong.*
> *May all beings live with ease.*

Sometimes I just say:

> *May all beings be happy.*
> *May all beings be free.*

This little practice helps me notice when I unwittingly layer suffering upon myself or cause difficulty to another person during the day. A friend told me, "The wish for all beings to be free sets the mind straight."

A vow shapes *how* we conduct the activities of our lives. It can apply equally to major tasks, such as raising children, and to minor tasks, like brushing our teeth. A vow may be especially useful for people who feel rudderless, such as the floater or the butterfly, and it comes easily to the moralist, who strives to do the right thing, or the perfectionist, who sets high standards. The latter two groups can help balance their zeal by formulating a *gentle* vow, like "compassion first."

A vow is the easiest of all meditations. We frontload all the work when we decide *what* we want our lives to stand for and then simply restate the vow occasionally to ourselves. If the vow truly reflects your heart's desire, it will have a power all its own, shaping your thoughts, feelings, and actions (see "The Power of Commitment" in Chapter 9).

As we progress on the path of self-compassion, the distinction between our own suffering and the suffering of others begins to blur. That is, as we stop fighting against personal pain, our attention naturally shifts to others. Compassion itself becomes the vow.

This impulse is behind one of the Dalai Lama's favorite vows, originally written by Shantideva, an Indian Buddhist monk from the 8th century CE:

> *For as long as space endures,*
> *And for as long as living beings remain,*
> *Until then may I, too, abide*
> *To dispel the misery of the world.*

APPENDIX C

further reading and practice

N ow that you've had a taste of self-compassion, the following resources can assist you in deepening your practice. Study is an important component of practice insofar as good ideas can inspire you and help you avoid unnecessary confusion. The books listed below explore compassion and mindfulness from a variety of angles, especially the intersection of modern psychology, Buddhist psychology, and psychotherapy. Many of the following materials don't focus *explicitly* on self-compassion, but they contain the spirit of the practice. Use them as an opportunity to experiment on your own. Some books below are written for a general audience and others are oriented more for mental health professionals, so please check online for reviews of books that may interest you.

There's no substitute for practicing under the guidance of a qualified teacher. Since many practitioners don't have access to teachers, audiovisual materials can be a valuable aid to practice. Some guided meditation tapes are listed below, as well as websites where information and other resources can be found.

Retreats are also an important part of deeper practice. Meditation training centers from the insight meditation (metta), Tibetan Buddhist (tonglen), and Zen (compassionate awareness) traditions are listed below.

BOOKS

Compassion

Brach, T. (2003). *Radical acceptance: Embracing your life with the heart of a Buddha.* New York: Bantam Dell.

Brown, B. (2010). *The gifts of imperfection: Let go of who you think you are supposed to be and embrace who you are.* Center City, MN: Hazeldon.

Chödrön, P. (1997). *When things fall apart: Heart advice for difficult times.* Boston: Shambhala.

Dalai Lama (2001). *An open heart: Practicing compassion in everyday life.* New York: Little, Brown.

Feldman, C. (2005). *Compassion: Listening to the cries of the world.* Berkeley, CA: Rodmell Press.

Flowers, S., & Stahl, B. (2011). *Living with your heart wide open: How mindfulness and compassion can free you from unworthiness, inadequacy, and shame.* Oakland, CA: New Harbinger Publications.

Fredrickson, B. (2013). *Love 2.0: Finding happiness and health in moments of connection.* New York: Plume.

Gilbert, P. (2009). *The compassionate mind: A new approach to life's challenges.* London: Constable & Robinson.

Gilbert, P., & Choden, (2014). *Mindful compassion: How the science of compassion can help you understand your emotions, live in the present, and connect deeply with others.* Oakland, CA: New Harbinger Publications

Goleman, D. (Ed.). (2003). *Healing emotions: Conversations with the Dalai Lama on mindfulness, emotions, and health.* Boston: Shambhala.

Hanh, T. N. (1998). *Teachings on love.* Berkeley, CA: Parallax Press.

Kolts, R., & Chodron, T. (2013). *Living with an open heart: How to cultivate compassion in everyday life.* London: Robinson Publishing.

Kornfield, J. (2009). *The wise heart: A guide to the universal teachings of Buddhist psychology.* New York: Bantam Books.

Makransky, J. (2007). *Awakening through love: Unveiling your deepest goodness.* Somerville, MA: Wisdom.

Neff, K. (2011). *Self-compassion: The proven power of being kind to yourself.* New York: William Morrow.

Salzberg, S. (1995). *Lovingkindness: The revolutionary art of happiness.* Boston: Shambhala.

Singer, T., & Bolz, M. (Eds.). (2013). *Compassion: Bridging practice and sci-*

ence. Leipzig, Germany: Max–Planck Institute. Free ebook available at *http://www.compassion-training.org/.*

Mindfulness

Baer, R. (2014). *Practising happiness: How mindfulness can free you from psychological traps and help you build the life you want.* London: Robinson.

Brach, T. (2013). *True refuge: Finding peace and freedom in your own awakened heart.* New York: Bantam Books.

Goldstein, J. (2013). *Mindfulness: A practical guide to awakening.* Louisville, CO: Sounds True.

Goldstein, J., & Kornfield, J. (1987). *Seeking the heart of wisdom: The path of insight meditation.* Boston: Shambhala.

Graham, L. (2013). *Bouncing back: Rewiring your brain for maximum resilience and well-being.* Novato, CA: New World Library.

Gunaratana, B. (2002). *Mindfulness in plain English.* Somerville, MA: Wisdom.

Hanh, T. N. (1976). *The miracle of mindfulness.* Boston: Beacon Press.

Hanson, R. (2009). *The Buddha's brain: The practical neuroscience of happiness, love, and wisdom.* Oakland, CA: New Harbinger Press.

Hanson, R. (2013). *Hardwiring happiness: The new brain science of contentment, calm, and confidence.* Easton, PA: Harmony Press.

Kabat-Zinn, J. (1990). *Full catastrophe living: Using the wisdom of your body and mind to face stress, pain, and illness.* New York: Dell.

Kabat-Zinn, J. (2011). *Mindfulness for beginners: Reclaiming the present moment—and your life.* Louisville, CO: Sounds True.

Kornfield, J. (2008). *The wise heart: A guide to the universal teachings of Buddhist psychology.* New York: Bantam Dell.

Magid, B. (2008). *Ending the pursuit of happiness: A Zen guide.* Somerville, MA: Wisdom.

Moffitt, P. (2008). *Dancing with life: Buddhist insights for finding meaning and joy in the face of suffering.* New York: Rodale Books.

Olendzki, A. (2010). *Unlimiting mind: The radically experiential psychology of Buddhism.* Somerville, MA: Wisdom Publications.

Salzberg, S. (2010). *Real happiness: The power of meditation: A 28-day program.* New York: Workman Publishing Company.

Stahl, B., & Goldstein, E. (2010). *A mindfulness-based stress reduction workbook.* Oakland, CA: New Harbinger Publications.

Teasdale, J., Williams, M., & Segal, Z. (2014). *The mindful way workbook:*

An 8-week program to free yourself from depression and emotional distress. New York: Guilford Press.

Tolle, E. (1999). *The power of now.* Novato, CA: New World Library.

Willard, C. (2010). *The child's mind: Mindfulness practices to help our children be more focused, calm, and relaxed.* Berkeley, CA: Parallax Press.

Psychotherapy

Brown, B. (1999). *Soul without shame: A guide to liberating yourself from the judge within.* Boston: Shambhala.

Geller, S., & Greenberg, L. (2011). *Therapeutic presence: A mindful approach to affective therapy.* Washington, DC: American Psychological Association Press.

Germer, C., & Siegel, R. (Eds.). (2012). *Wisdom and compassion in psychotherapy: Deepening mindfulness in clinical practice.* New York: Guilford Press.

Germer, C., Siegel, R., & Fulton, P. (Eds.). (2013). *Mindfulness and psychotherapy, second edition.* New York: Guilford Press.

Gilbert, P. (2010). *Compassion focused therapy: Distinctive features.* London: Routledge.

Hayes, S., & Smith, S. (2005). *Get out of your mind and into your life: The new acceptance and commitment therapy.* Oakland, CA: New Harbinger.

Hayes, S., Strosahl, K., & Wilson, K. (2011). *Acceptance and commitment therapy: The process and practice of mindful change, second edition.* New York: Guilford Press.

Harris, R., & Hayes, S. (2009). *ACT made simple: An easy-to-read primer on acceptance and commitment therapy.* Oakland, CA: New Harbinger Publications.

Kolts, R. (2013). *The compassionate-mind guide to managing your anger: Using compassion-focused therapy to calm your rage and heal your relationships.* Oakland, CA: New Harbinger Press.

Ladner, L. (2004). *The lost art of compassion: Discovering the practice of happiness in the meeting of Buddhism and psychology.* New York: HarperCollins.

Orsillo, S., & Roemer, L. (2011). *The mindful way through anxiety: Break free from chronic worry and reclaim your life.* New York: Guilford Press.

Pollak, S., Pedulla, T., & Siegel, R. (2014). *Sitting together: Essential skills for mindfulness-based psychotherapy.* New York: Guilford Press.

Segal, Z., Williams, M., & Teasdale, J. (2012). *Mindfulness-based cognitive therapy for depression, second edition.* New York: Guilford Press.

Siegel, D. (2010). *Mindsight: The new science of personal transformation.* New York: Bantam Books.

Siegel, R. (2009). *The mindfulness solution: Everyday practices for everyday problems.* New York: Guilford Press.

Tirch, D. (2012). *The compassionate-mind guide to overcoming anxiety: Using compassion focused therapy to calm worry, panic, and fear.* Oakland, CA: New Harbinger Press.

Williams, M., Teasdale, J., & Segal, Z. (2007). *The mindful way through depression: Freeing yourself from chronic unhappiness.* New York: Guilford Press.

Welford, M. (2013). *The power of self-compassion: Using compassion-focused therapy to end self-criticism and build self-confidence.* Oakland, CA: New Harbinger Press.

WEBSITES

Author information and guided self-compassion meditations: *www.MindfulSelfCompassion.org*

Online group on loving-kindness: *groups.yahoo.com/group/giftoflovingkindness*

Self-compassion research: *www.self-compassion.org*

Science of meditation and compassion: *www.mindandlife.org*

Teachers:
 Tara Brach: *www.tarabrach.com*
 Pema Chödrön: *www.shambhala.org/teachers/pema/*
 Dalai Lama: *www.dalailama.com*
 Jon Kabat-Zinn : *www.umassmed.edu/cfm/index.aspx*
 Jack Kornfield: *www.jackkornfield.org*
 Lama Surya Das: *www.dzogchen.org*
 Sharon Salzberg: *www.sharonsalzberg.com*
 Thich Nhat Hanh: *www.iamhome.org, www.plumvillage.org*

Buddhist practice journals: *www.tricycle.com, www.thebuddhadharma.com, www.shambhalasun.com*

Mindfulness-based stress reduction: *www.umassmed.edu/cfm*

Mindfulness and psychotherapy: *www.meditationandpsychotherapy.org*

GUIDED MEDITATION AND TEACHING

Audiovisual materials of all kinds: *www.soundstrue.com*

Recommended guided meditation from Sounds True:

- Tara Brach (2014). *Developing Self-Compassion.*
- Tara Brach (2005). *Radical Self-Acceptance: A Buddhist Guide to Freeing Yourself from Shame.*
- Tara Brach (2009). *Meditations for Emotional Healing: Finding Freedom in the Face of Difficulty.*
- Jack Kornfield (2011). *Guided Meditations for Self-Healing: Essential Practices to Relieve Physical and Emotional Suffering and Enhance Recovery.*
- Jack Kornfield (2014). *The Healing Power of Love.*
- Jon Kabat-Zinn (2006). *Mindfulness for Beginners: Explore the Infinite Potential that Lies Within This Very Moment.*
- Joseph Goldstein (2013). *Mindfulness: Six Guided Practices for Awakening.* Essential mindfulness meditations complement the teachings in the book of the same title.
- Kristin Neff (2013). *Self-Compassion Step by Step: The Proven Power of Being Kind to Yourself.*
- Pema Chödrön (2012). *Awakening Love: Teachings and Practices to Cultivate a Limitless Heart.* Pema Chödrön shows us how to shed our emotional armor and open ourselves to limitless love.
- Rick Hanson (2012). *The Compassionate Brain: Activating the Neural Circuits of Kindness, Caring, and Love.*
- Sharon Salzberg (2004). *Lovingkindness Meditation: Learning to Love Through Insight Meditation.*
- Sharon Salzberg (2009). *Guided Meditations for Love and Wisdom.*
- Sharon Salzberg and Joseph Goldstein (2011). *Insight Meditation: An In-Depth Course on How to Meditate.*

Talks from insight meditation retreats (free downloads):
www.dharmaseed.org

Guided mindfulness meditation CDs by Jon Kabat-Zinn:
www.mindfulnesscds.com

Guided meditation and teaching by Pema Chödrön:
www.pemachodrontapes.org

MEDITATION TRAINING

Depending on the teacher, self-compassion is integrated into meditation training to varying degrees. Before you take instruction or go on a retreat, please research your teacher very carefully to determine whether his or her teaching style is compatible with your needs.

To start your search for meditation centers and communities in your area, go to *www.dharma.org/ims/mr_links.html* and click on outside resources.

For a broad listing of Buddhist meditation centers around the world, go to *www.buddhanet.info/wbd/* and click on outside resources.

The following meditation centers are likely to have teaching and meditation programs that are compatible with the material presented in this book:

United States

Non-Buddhist

Center for Mindfulness in Medicine, Health, and Society
55 Lake Avenue North
Worcester, MA 01655
www.umassmed.edu/cfm

Insight Meditation Tradition

Barre Center for Buddhist Studies
149 Lockwood Road
Barre, MA 01005
www.dharma.org/bcbs

Bhavana Society
97 Meditation Trail
High View, WV 26808
www.bhavanasociety.org

Cambridge Insight Meditation Center
331 Broadway
Cambridge, MA 02139
www.cimc.info

InsightLA
1430 Olympic Boulevard
Santa Monica, CA 90404
www.insightla.org

Insight Meditation Community of Washington, D.C.
P.O. Box 3
Cabin John, MD 20818
www.imcw.org

Insight Meditation Society
1230 Pleasant Street
Barre, MA 01005
www.dharma.org/ims

Metta Forest Monastery
13560 Muutama Lane
Valley Center, CA 92082
www.watmetta.org

Mid-America Dharma
455 East 80th Terrace
Kansas City, MO 64131
www.midamericadharma.org

New York Insight Meditation Center
28 West 27th Street, 10th floor
New York, NY 10001
www.nyimc.org

Spirit Rock Meditation Center
P.O. Box 169
Woodacre, CA 94973
www.spiritrock.org

Zen Tradition

Blue Cliff Monastery
3 Mindfulness Road
Pine Bush, NY 12566
www.bluecliffmonastery.org

Boundless Way Zen
Greater Boston Zen Center
288 Norfolk St.,
Cambridge, MA 02139
www.boundlesswayzen.org

Deer Park Monastery
2499 Melru Lane
Escondido, CA 92026
www.deerparkmonastery.org

Upaya Zen Center
1404 Cerro Gordo Road
Santa Fe, NM 87501
www.upaya.org

Village Zendo
588 Broadway, Suite 1108
New York, NY 10012-5238
villagezendo.org

Zen Center of San Diego
2047 Feldspar Street
San Diego, CA 92109-3551
www.zencentersandiego.org

Tibetan Buddhist Tradition

Dzogchen Foundation
For teaching and retreat schedule, go to *www.dzogchen.org*.

Naropa University
2130 Arapahoe Avenue
Boulder, CO 80302
www.naropa.edu

Shambhala Mountain Center
151 Shambhala Way
Red Feather Lakes, CO 80545
www.shambhalamountain.org

Tenzin Gyatso Institute for Wisdom and Compassion
165 Game Farm Road
Berne, NY 12023
www.tenzingyatsoinstitute.org.

Canada

Gampo Abbey
Pleasant Bay
Cape Brenton, NS BOE 2PO
Canada
www.gampoabbey.org

For other Canadian meditation centers, go to *www.gosit.org.*

Europe

Non-Buddhist

Centre for Mindfulness Research and Practice
School of Psychology
Dean Street Building
Bangor University
Bangor LL57 1UT
UK
www.bangor.ac.uk/mindfulness

Insight Meditation Tradition

Gaia House
West Ogwell, Newton Abbot
Devon TQ12 6EW
UK
www.gaiahouse.co.uk

Kalyana Centre
Eva Bruha
40 John Street Dingle
County Kerry
Ireland
www.kalyanacentre.com

Meditationszentrum Beatenberg
Waldegg
Beatenberg CH-3803
Switzerland
www.karuna.ch

Seminarhaus Engl
Engl 1

Unterdietfurt 84339

Bavaria

Germany

www.seminarhaus-engl.de

For other European centers, go to *www.mahasi.eu/centers.html*

Zen Tradition

Plum Village Practice Center

13 Martineau

Dieulivol 33580

France

www.plumvillage.org

Tibetan Buddhist Tradition

Shambhala Europe

Kartäuserwall 20

Köln 50678

Germany

shambhala-europe.org

For Shambhala centers worldwide, go to *www.shambhala.org/centers.*

Sanctuary of Enlightened Action

Lerab Ling

L'Engayresque

34650 Roquerdonde

France

www.lerabling.org

Australia/New Zealand

Insight Meditation Tradition

Bodhinyanarama Monastery
17 Rakau Grove, Stokes Valley
Lower Hutt 5019
New Zealand
www.bodhinyanarama.net.nz/

Santi Forest Monastery
100 Coalmines Road
Bundanoon
New South Wales 2578
Australia
santifm.org/santi

For other Australian insight meditation centers, go to *www.dharma.org.au*.

For other New Zealand insight meditation centers, go to *www.insightmeditation.org.nz/wiki*.

Zen Tradition

For Zen centers in Australia, go to *iriz.hanazono.ac.jp/zen_centers/centers_ data/australi.htm*.

For Zen centers in New Zealand, go to *iriz.hanazono.ac.jp/zen_centers/ centers_data/newzeal.htm*.

Tibetan Buddhist Tradition

Shambhala Meditation Centre Auckland
Grey Lynn Community Centre
510 Richmond Road
Grey Lynn, Auckland
New Zealand
www.auckland.shambhala.info

notes

INTRODUCTION

40% of marriages end in divorce: Hurley, D. (2005, April 19). Divorce rate: It's not as high as you think. *New York Times,* Retrieved December 14, 2008, from *www.divorcereform.org/nyt05.html.* Kreider, R., & Fields, J. (2002, February). Number, timing, and duration of marriages and divorces: 1996, February. *U.S. Census Bureau Current Population Reports.*

[Compassion] is the state of wishing: Davidson, R., & Harrington, A. (2002). *Visions of compassion: Western scientists and Tibetan Buddhists examine human nature* (p. 98). Oxford, UK: Oxford University Press.

cultivate a new relationship to ourselves: Neff, K. D. (2003). Self-compassion: An alternative conceptualization of a healthy attitude toward oneself. *Self and Identity, 2,* 85–102.

most thoroughly researched of all psychotherapy methods: Walsh, R., & Shapiro, S. (2006). The meeting of meditative disciplines and Western psychology: A mutually enriching dialogue. *American Psychologist, 61*(3), 227–239.

awareness of present experience, with acceptance: Germer, C. (2005). Mindfulness: What is it? What does it matter? In C. Germer, R. Siegel, & P. Fulton (Eds.), *Mindfulness and psychotherapy* (pp. 3–27). New York: Guilford Press.

my father met a mountaineer: Harrer, H. (1953/1997). *Seven years in Tibet.* New York: Penguin Group (USA)/Tarcher.

introduced the Buddhist practice of mindfulness and compassion: Kabat-Zinn, J. (1990). *Full catastrophe living: Using the wisdom of your body and mind to face stress, pain, and illness.* New York: Dell.

CHAPTER 1. BEING KIND TO YOURSELF

it's the resentment against suffering that is the real pain: Ginsberg, A. (1997). In Smith, J. (Ed.), *Everyday mind* (p. 96). New York: Riverhead Books.

there's "no negation" in the unconscious mind: Freud, S. (1915/1971). The unconscious. In *The standard edition of the complete psychological works of Sigmund Freud* (Vol. 14, p. 186). London: Hogarth Press.

we typically return to our former level of happiness: Diener, E., Lucas, R., & Scollon, C. (2006). Beyond the hedonic treadmill: Revising the adaptation theory of well-being. *American Psychologist, 61*(4), 304–314.

The Hedonic Treadmill: Brickman, P., & Campbell, D. T. (1971). Hedonic relativism and planning the good society. In M. H. Appley (Ed.), *Adaptation level theory: A symposium* (pp. 287–302). New York: Academic Press.

How many hippos worry: Sapolsky, R. (2004). *Why zebras don't get ulcers: An updated guide to stress, stress related diseases, and coping* (p. 5). New York: Holt.

telomeres: Epel, E., Blackburn, E., Lin, J., Dhabhar, F., Adler, N., Morrow, J., & Cawthon, R. (2004). Accelerated telomere shortening in response to life stress. *Proceedings of the National Academy of Sciences, 101*(49), 17312–17315. Sapolsky, R. (2004). Organismal stress and telomeric aging: An unexpected connection. *Proceedings of the National Academy of Sciences, 101*(50), 17323–17324.

Embracing Misery in Marriage: Gehart, D., & McCollum, E. (2007). Engaging suffering: Towards a mindful re-visioning of family therapy practice. *Journal of Marital and Family Therapy, 33*(2), 214–226.

tracked 650 couples to discover what made marriages successful: Gottman, J. (1999). *The marriage clinic: A scientifically-based marital therapy.* New York: Norton. Gottman, J., Coan, J., Carrere, S., & Swanson, C. (1998). Predicting marital happiness and stability from newly wed interactions. *Journal of Marriage and the Family, 60,* 5–22. Gottman, J., & Silver, N. (1999). *The seven principles for making marriage work.* New York: Three Rivers Press.

acceptance-based couple therapy: Christensen, A., Atkins, D., Yi, J., Baucom, D., & George, W. (2006). Couple and individual adjustment for 2 years following a randomized clinical trial comparing traditional versus integrative behavioral couple therapy. *Journal of Consulting and Clinical Psychology, 74*(6), 1180–1191. Christensen, A., & Jacobson, N. (2000). *Reconcilable differences.* New York: Guilford Press. Jacobson,

N., & Christensen, A. (1996). *Acceptance and change in couple therapy: A therapist's guide to transforming relationships.* New York: Norton.

The Benefit of Worry: Borkovec, T., & Hu, S. (1990). The effect of worry on cardiovascular response to phobic imagery. *Behaviour Research and Therapy, 28*(1), 69–73.

affecting at least five million people: Agency for Health Care Policy and Research. (1994). *Acute low back problems in adults: Clinical practice guideline No. 14* (AHCPR Publication No. 95-0642). Rockville, MD: Public Health Service, U.S. Department of Health and Human Services.

60–70% of Americans get lower back pain: Hart, L., Deyo, R., & Cherkin, D. (1995). Physician office visits for low back pain: Frequency, clinical evaluation, and treatment patterns from a U.S. national survey. *Spine, 20*(1), 11–19. Van Tulder, M., Koes, B., & Bombardier, C. (2002). Low back pain. *Best Practice and Research in Clinical Rheumatology 16,* 761–775.

people *without* chronic back pain have the same structural back problems: Jensen, M., Brant-Zawadzki, M., Obucowski, N., Modic, M., Malkasian, D., & Ross, J. (1994). Magnetic resonance imaging of the lumbar spine in people without back pain. *New England Journal of Medicine, 331*(2), 69–73.

success rate of back surgery for herniated disks: Peul, W., van den Hout, W., Brand, R., Thomeer, R., Koes, B., et al. (2008). Prolonged conservative care versus early surgery in patients with sciatica caused by lumbar disc herniation: Two year results of a randomised controlled trial. *British Journal of Medicine, 336,* 1355–1358.

the most valuable treatment for a herniated disk: Siegel, R. (2005). In C. Germer, R. Siegel, & P. Fulton (Eds.), *Mindfulness and psychotherapy* (pp. 173–196). New York: Guilford Press. Siegel, R. D., Urdang, M., & Johnson, D. (2001). *Back sense: A revolutionary approach to halting the cycle of back pain.* New York: Broadway Books.

prevalence of chronic back pain is lowest in developing countries: Volinn, E. (1997). The epidemiology of low back pain in the rest of the world: A review of surveys in low middle income countries. *Spine, 22*(15), 1747–1754.

Job Dissatisfaction Predicts Chronic Low Back Pain: Williams, R., Pruitt, S., Doctor, J., Epping-Jordan, J., Wahlgren, D., Grant, I., et al. (1998). The contribution of job satisfaction to the transition from acute to chronic low back pain. *Archives of Physical Medicine and Rehabilitation, 79*(4), 366–374.

reports having insomnia in any given year: Becker, P. (2006). Insomnia: Prevalence, impact, pathogenesis, differential diagnosis, and evaluation. *Psychiatric Clinics of North America, 29*(4), 855–870.

trying too hard to fall asleep: Lundh, L. (2005). Role of acceptance and mindfulness in the treatment of insomnia. *Journal of Cognitive Psychotherapy: An International Quarterly, 19*(1), 29–39.

you're better off in the casket than doing the eulogy: Seinfeld, J. (2008, September 19). Thinkexist: Jerry Seinfeld quotes. *thinkexist.com/quotes/Jerry_Seinfeld.*

at least a third of us feel that our anxiety is "excessive": Stein, M., Walker, J., & Forde, D. (1996). Public-speaking fears in a community sample: Prevalence, impact on functioning, and diagnostic classification. *Archives of General Psychiatry, 53*(2), 169–174.

Suppress It!: Wegner, D., Schneider, D., Carter, S., & White, T. (1987). Paradoxical effects of thought suppression. *Journal of Personality and Social Psychology, 53*(1), 5–13.

on *emotional* suppression: Gailliot, M., Baumeister, R., DeWall, C., Maner, J., Plant, E., Tice, D., et al. (2007). Self-control relies on glucose as a limited energy source: Willpower is more than a metaphor. *Journal of Personality and Social Psychology, 92*(2), 325–336.

Suzanne and Michael were going through "cold hell": Germer, C. (2006, Spring). Getting along: Loving the other without losing yourself. *Tricycle: The Buddhist Review,* pp. 25–27.

able to reduce their medication: Kuyken, W., Byford, S., Taylor, R., Watkins, E., Holden, E., White, K., et al. (2008). Mindfulness-based cognitive therapy to prevent relapse in recurrent depression. *Journal of Consulting and Clinical Psychology, 76*(6), 966–978.

if you can't be fully present with the difficult moments: Moffitt, P. (2008). *Dancing with life: Buddhist insights for finding meaning and joy in the face of suffering* (p. 41). New York: Rodale Press.

it's the process of establishing a new *relationship* with our thoughts: Longmore, R., & Worrell, M. (2007). Do we need to challenge thoughts in cognitive behavior therapy? *Clinical Psychology Review, 27*(2), 173–187. Hayes, S., Follette, V., & Linehan, M. (Eds.). (2004). *Mindfulness and acceptance: Expanding the cognitive–behavioral tradition.* New York: Guilford Press. Roemer, L., & Orsillo, S. (2009). *Mindfulness- and acceptance-based behavioral therapies in practice.* New York: Guilford Press.

the Latin roots *com* (with) *pati* (suffer): Online Etymology Dictionary. Retrieved September 20, 2008, from *www.etymonline.com/index.php?term=compassion.*

CHAPTER 2. LISTENING TO YOUR BODY

It is just simple attention: Feldman, C., & Kornfield, J. (1991). *Stories of the spirit, stories of the heart* (p. 83). New York: HarperCollins.

Big Dipper: Goldstein, J. (1993). *Insight meditation: The practice of freedom* (p. 112). Boston: Shambhala.

Mary Oliver reminds us in this poem: Oliver, M. (2005). "Mindful." In *Why I wake early: New poems* (pp. 58–59). Boston: Beacon Press.

"Knowing what you are experiencing *while* you're experiencing it": Armstrong, G. (2008, January 9). From a talk at the Mind and Life Institute Scientist's Retreat, Insight Meditation Society, Barre, MA.

Suddenly the city: Bamber, L. (2008). "Suddenly the city." In *Metropolitan Tang* (p. 27). Jaffrey, NH: Black Sparrow.

The "Default Network": Gusnard, D., & Raichle, M. (2001). Searching for a baseline: Functional imaging and the resting human brain. *Nature Reviews/Neuroscience, 2,* 685–694.

Default network during meditation using fMRI: Pagnoni, G., Cekic, M., & Guo, Y. (2008). "Thinking about not-thinking": Neural correlates of conceptual processing during Zen meditation. *PLoS ONE, 3*(9). *www.plosone.org/article/info%3Adoi%2F10.1371%2Fjournal.pone.0003083.*

There are two categories of mindfulness meditation: Kabat-Zinn, J. (1990). *Full catastrophe living: Using the wisdom of your body and mind to face stress, pain, and illness.* New York: Dell.

the freedom to "respond" rather than "react": Kabat-Zinn, J. (1990). *Full catastrophe living: Using the wisdom of your body and mind to face stress, pain, and illness* (pp. 264–273). New York: Dell.

Training Your Brain: Davidson, R. J., Kabat-Zinn, J., Schumacher, J., Rosenkranz, M., Muller, D., Santorelli, S., et al. (2003). Alterations in brain and immune function produced by mindfulness meditation. *Psychosomatic Medicine, 65*(4), 564–570.

impact of the MBSR program on immune functioning: Myers, H., & Creswell, D. (2008). Mindfulness meditation slows progression of HIV, study suggests. *ScienceDaily.* Retrieved July 28, 2008, from *www.sciencedaily.com/releases/2008/07/080724215644. htm.*

interleukin-6: Pace, T., Negi, L., Adame, D., Cole, S., Sivilli, T., Brown, T. L, Issa, M., & Raison, C. (2008). Effect of compassion meditation on neuroendocrine, innate immune and behavioral responses to psychosocial stress. *Psychoneuroimmunology,* doi:10.1016/j.psyneuen.2008.08.011.

parts of the brain even grow thicker: Lazar, S., Kerr, C., Wasserman, R., Gray, J., Greve, D., Treadway, M., et al. (2005). Meditation experience is associated with increased cortical thickness. *NeuroReport, 16*(17), 1893–1897.

What Mindfulness Is Not: Bhikkhu, T. (2008, Summer). Mindfulness defined: Street smarts for the path. *Insight Journal* (Barre Center for Buddhist Studies; pp. 11–15). Olendzki, A. (2008, Fall). The real practice of mindfulness. *Buddhadharma: The Practitioner's Quarterly* (pp. 50–57). Siegel, R., Germer, C., & Olendzki, A. (2008).

Mindfulness: What is it? Where did it come from? In F. Didonna (Ed.), *Clinical handbook of mindfulness* (pp. 17–35). New York: Springer.

the power of brief mindfulness exercises: Singh, N., Wahler, R., Adkins, A., & Myers, R. (2003). Soles of the feet: A mindfulness-based self-control intervention for aggression by an individual with mild mental retardation and mental illness. *Research in Developmental Disabilities, 24*(3), 158–169.

CHAPTER 3. BRINGING IN DIFFICULT EMOTIONS

How can emotions not be part of that singing life: Hirshfield, J. (1997). In J. Smith (Ed.), *Everyday mind* (p. 46). New York: Riverhead Books.

How We Create Suffering: Mindfulness is bottom-up processing, starting with simple sensation. See Siegel, R., Germer, C., & Olendzki, A. (2009). Mindfulness: What is it? Where did it come from? In F. Didonna (Ed.), *Clinical handbook of mindfulness* (p. 32) New York: Springer. Hart, W. (1987). *The art of living: Vipassana meditation: As taught by S. N. Goenka.* San Francisco: HarperCollins. Full quote (p. 97): "A sensation appears, and liking or disliking begins. This fleeting moment, if we are unaware of it, is repeated and intensified into craving and aversion, becoming a strong emotion that eventually overpowers the conscious mind. We become caught up in the emotion, and all our better judgment is swept aside. The result is that we find ourselves engaged in unwholesome speech and action, harming ourselves and others. We create misery for ourselves, suffering now and in the future, because of one moment of blind reaction."

Do We Have Free Will?: Libet, B. (1999). Do we have free will? In B. Libet, A. Freeman, & K. Sutherland (Eds.), *The volitional brain: Towards a neuroscience of free will* (pp. 47–57). Thorverton, UK: Imprint Academic.

"Noting" is an umbrella term: See Young, S. (2006, October 16). *How to note and label.* Retrieved September 24, 2008, from *www.shinzen.org/Retreat%20Reading/How%20to%20Note%20and%20Label.pdf.*

How does mindfulness meditation actually help balance our emotions?: Creswell, D., Way, B., Eisenberger, N., & Lieberman, M. (2007). Neural correlates of dispositional mindfulness during affect labeling. *Psychosomatic Medicine, 69*(6), 560–565.

one set of basic emotions over any other: Ortony, A., & Turner, T. J. (1990). What's basic about basic emotions? *Psychological Review, 97,* 315–331.

comprehensive list of emotion words: DeRose, S. (2005, July 6). *The compass DeRose guide to emotion words.* Retrieved September 24, 2008, from *www.derose.net/steve/resources/emotionwords/ewords.html.*

Over 50% of people in the United States have experienced trauma: Kessler, R., Sonnega, A., Bromet, E., Hughes, M., & Nelson, C. (1995). Posttraumatic stress disorder in the National Comorbidity Survey. *Archives of General Psychiatry, 52*(12), 1048–1060.

sexually abused as children: Dube, S., Anda, R., Whitfield, C., Brown, D., Felitti, V., Dong, M., et al. (2005). Long-term consequences of childhood sexual abuse by gender of victim. *American Journal of Preventive Medicine, 28*(5), 430–438. Finkelhor, D. (1994). Current information on the scope and nature of child sexual abuse. *The Future of Children, 4*(2), 31–53. Gorey, K., & Leslie, D. (1997). The prevalence of child sexual abuse: Integrative review adjustment for potential response and measurement biases. *Child Abuse and Neglect, 21*(4), 391–398.

CHAPTER 4. WHAT'S SELF-COMPASSION?

Before you know kindness as the deepest thing inside: Nye, N. (1995). Kindness. In *Words under the words* (pp. 42–43). Portland, OR: Eighth Mountain Press.

Loving-kindness is wishing *happiness* for another person: Dalai Lama & Vreeland, N. (2001). *An open heart: Practicing compassion in everyday life* (p. 96). New York: Little, Brown.

"the heart quivers in response": Silberman, S. (2008, January). Because life is difficult, the only choice is kindness (an interview with Sylvia Boorstein). *Shambhala Sun,* p. 69.

Self-Compassion Scale: Neff, K. D. (2003). Development and validation of a scale to measure self-compassion. *Self and Identity, 2,* 223–250. Neff, K. D. (2004). Self-compassion and psychological well-being. *Constructivism in the Human Sciences, 9,* 27–37.

the wish to be happy and free from suffering: Dalai Lama. (2001). *An open heart: Practicing compassion in everyday life* (p. 30). New York: Little, Brown. H. H. Dalai Lama wrote: "The purpose of spiritual practice is to fulfill our desire for happiness. We are all equal in wishing to be happy and to overcome our suffering, and I believe we all share the right to fulfill this aspiration."

"tend and befriend": Taylor, S. (2006). Tend and befriend: Biobehavioral bases of affiliation under stress. *Current Directions in Psychological Science, 15*(6), 273–277. Taylor, S. (2002). *The tending instinct: How nurturing is essential to who we are and how we live.* New York: Times Books.

the area of the brain called the *insula*: Blakeslee, S. (2007, February 6). A small part of the brain, and its profound effects. *New York Times/Mental Health and Behavior.* Retrieved September 24, 2008, from *www.nytimes.com/2007/02/06/health/psychology/06brain.html?_r=1&scp=1&sq=Blakeslee%20A%20small%20part%20of%20the%20brain&st.*

people high in empathy had more gray matter: Blakeslee, S., & Blakeslee, M. (2007, August–September). Where body and mind meet. *Scientific American Mind,* pp. 44–51. Critchley, H. (2005). Neural mechanisms of autonomic, affective, and cognitive integration. *Journal of Comparative Neurology, 493,* 154–166. Critchley, H., Wiens, S., Rotshstein, P., Öhman, A., & Dolan, R. (2004). Neural systems supporting interoceptive awareness. *Nature Neuroscience, 7,* 189–195.

mindfulness-based stress reduction: Kabat-Zinn, J. (1990). *Full catastrophe living: Using the wisdom of your body and mind to face stress, pain, and illness.* New York: Dell.

sensations enter the rear part of the insula: Craig, A. (2003). Interoception: The sense of the physiological condition of the body. *Current Opinion in Neurobiology, 13,* 500–505.

increases in self-compassion were found after training: Shapiro, S., Brown, K., & Biegel, G. (2007). Teaching self-care to caregivers: Effects of mindfulness-based stress reduction on the mental health of therapists in training. *Training and Education in Professional Psychology, 1*(2), 105–115.

This being human is a guest house: Barks, C., & Moyne, J. (1997). The guest house. In *The Essential Rumi* (p. 109). San Francisco: Harper.

18 personal "schemas": Young, J., Klosko, J., & Weishaar, M. (2003). *Schema therapy: A practitioner's guide* (pp. 14–17). New York: Guilford Press.

working mindfully and compassionately with our schemas: Bennett-Goleman, T. (2001). *Emotional alchemy.* New York: Harmony Books.

"orchestra without a conductor": Singer, W. (2005, November 10). Lecture presented at the Mind and Life Institute Conference, The Science and Clinical Applications of Meditation, Washington, DC.

a careful look at our mental activity: Fulton, P. R. (2008). *Anatta*: Self, non-self, and the therapist. In S. F. Hick & T. Bien (Eds.), *Mindfulness and the therapeutic relationship* (pp. 55-71). New York: Guilford Press.

"compassion directed toward oneself is humility": Weil, S. (1998). In E. Springsted (Ed.), *Selected writings* (p. 143). Maryknoll, NY: Orbis Books.

What Does the Research Show?: Neff, K. D. (2008). Self-compassion: Moving beyond the pitfalls of a separate self-concept. In J. Bauer & H. A. Wayment (Eds.), *Transcending self-interest: Psychological explorations of the quiet ego.* Washington DC: APA Books.

softens the impact of negative events in our lives: Leary, M. R., Tate, E. B., Adams, C. E., Allen, A. B., & Hancock, J. (2007). Self-compassion and reactions to unpleasant self-relevant events: The implications of treating oneself kindly. *Journal of Personality and Social Psychology, 92,* 887–904.

when a self-compassionate person experiences academic failure: Neff, K. D., Hseih, Y., & Dejitthirat, K. (2005). Self-compassion, achievement goals, and coping with academic failure. *Self and Identity, 4,* 263–287.

self-esteem is not particularly related to how others evaluate them: Neff, K. D., Kirkpatrick, K., & Rude, S. S. (2007). Self-compassion and its link to adaptive psychological functioning. *Journal of Research in Personality, 41,* 139–154. Neff, K. D., & Vonk, R. (in press). Self-compassion versus global self-esteem: Two different ways of relating to oneself. *Journal of Personality.*

self-compassion isn't related to narcissism: Webster, D., & Kruglanski, A. (1994). Individual differences in need for cognitive closure. *Journal of Personality and Social Psychology, 67,* 1049–1062.

Dieting through Self-Compassion: Adams, C., & Leary, M. (2007). Promoting self-compassionate attitudes toward eating among restrictive and guilty eaters. *Journal of Social and Clinical Psychology, 26*(10), 1120–1144.

more strongly than scores on a mindfulness scale: Neff, K. (2008, April 16). *Self-compassion, mindfulness, and psychological health.* Paper presented at the 6th Annual International Scientific Conference for Clinicians, Researchers, and Educators, Worcester, MA.

self-compassion predicts psychological well-being: Neff, K., Rude, S., & Kirkpatrick, K. (2007). An examination of self-compassion in relation to positive psychological functioning and personality traits. *Journal of Research in Personality, 41,* 908–916.

compassionate mind training: Gilbert, P., & Procter, S. (2006). Compassionate mind training for people with high shame and self-criticism: Overview and pilot study of a group therapy approach. *Clinical Psychology and Psychotherapy, 13,* 353–379.

the future of self-compassion research is promising and bright: Preliminary investigations into a wide range of clinical conditions include: Thompson, B. & Waltz, J. (2008). Self-compassion and PTSD symptom severity. *Journal of Traumatic Stress, 21*(6), 556–558. Johnson, D., Penn, D., Fredrickson, B., Meyer, P., Kring, A., & Brantley, M. (2009). Loving-kindness meditation to enhance recovery from negative symptoms of schizophrenia. *Journal of Clinical Psychology.* Published online March 6, 2009, in session 65, 1–11.

CHAPTER 5. PATHWAYS TO SELF-COMPASSION

The time will come: Walcott, D. (1987). Love after love. In *Derek Walcott: Collected poems, 1948–1984* (p. 328). New York: Farrar, Straus and Giroux.

Warm Hands, Warm Heart: Williams, L., & Bargh, J. (2008). Experiencing physical warmth promotes interpersonal warmth. *Science, 322*(5901), 606–607.

The brain comprises only 2% of our body weight: Russell, P. (1979). *The brain book: Know your own mind and how to use it* (p. 67). New York: Routledge.

"creative hopelessness": Hayes, S. (2004). Acceptance and Commitment Therapy and the new behavior therapies: Mindfulness, acceptance and relationship. In

S. Hayes, V. Follette, & M. Linehan (Eds.), *Mindfulness and acceptance: Expanding the cognitive-behavioral tradition* (p. 18). New York: Guilford Press.

enjoyable activities can help: For a list of adult pleasant events, see pages 157–159 of: Linehan, M. (1993). *Skills training manual for treating borderline personality disorder.* New York: Guilford Press.

"wisely selfish": Dalai Lama & Hopkins, J. (2002). *How to practice: The way to a meaningful life* (pp. 80–81). New York: Atria Books.

Spending Money on Others: Dunn, E., Aknin, L., & Norton, M. (2008). Spending money on others promotes happiness. *Science, 319*(5870), 1687–1688.

The merciful man does himself good: *New American Standard Bible.* (1997). Proverbs 11:17. La Habra, CA: Foundation Publications.

On traversing all directions with the mind: Ireland, J. (1997). *"Udana" and the "Itivattaka": Two classics from the Pali Canon* (p. 62). Kandy, Sri Lanka: Buddhist Publication Society.

as they love their own bodies: *International Standard Version, New Testament.* (1998). Ephesians 5:28. Fullerton, CA: Davidson Press.

Savoring **refers to:** Bryant, R., & Veroff, J. (2007). *Savoring: A new model of positive experience* (p. xi). Mahwah, NJ: Erlbaum.

I can wade Grief—: Dickinson, E. (1995). I can wade grief. In J. Parini (Ed.), *The Columbia University anthology of American poetry* (p. 250). New York: Columbia University Press.

Research has shown that the savoring of pleasant experiences: Bryant, R., & Veroff, J. (2007). *Savoring: A new model of positive experience* (pp. 198–215). Mahwah, NJ: Erlbaum.

Interventions for Happiness: Seligman, M., Rashid, T., & Parks, A. (2006). Positive psychotherapy. *American Psychologist, 61*(8), 774–788.

What Are Positive Emotions?: Lewis, M., Haviland-Jones, J., & Barrett, L. (2008). *Handbook of emotions* (3rd ed.). New York: Guilford Press.

A review of over 225 published papers: Lyubomirsky, S., King, L., & Diener, E. (2005). The benefits of frequent positive affect: Does happiness lead to success? *Psychological Bulletin, 131*(6), 803–855. Mobini, S., & Grant, A. (2007). Clinical implications of attentional bias in anxiety disorders: An integrative literature review. *Psychotherapy: Theory, Research, Practice, Training, 44,* 450–462.

The Emotional Brain: Miller, C. (2008, September 22). Sad brain, happy brain. *Time,* pp. 51, 52, 56. Harrison, N., & Critchley, H. (2007). Affective neuroscience and psychiatry. *British Journal of Psychiatry, 191,* 192–194. Davidson, R. (2003). Affective neuroscience and psychophysiology: Toward a synthesis. *Psychophysiology, 40,*

655–665. Phan, K., Wagner, T., Taylor, S., & Liberzon, I. (2002). Functional neuro-anatomy of emotion: A meta-analysis of emotion activation studies in PET and fMRI. *Neuroimage, 16*(2), 331–348.

Reptiles have rudimentary elements of the limbic system: Konner, M. (2003). *The tangled wing: Biological constraints on the human spirit.* New York: Macmillan.

college yearbook photographs: Harker, L., & Keltner, D. (2001). Expression of positive emotion in women's college yearbook pictures and their relationship to personality and life outcomes across adulthood. *Journal of Personality and Social Psychology, 80*(1), 112–124.

Catholic nuns: Danner, D., Snowdon, D., & Friesen, W. (2001). Positive emotions in early life and longevity: Findings from the Nun Study. *Journal of Personality and Social Psychology, 80*(5), 804–813.

positive emotions allow us to see the big picture: Fredrickson, B. (2004). The broaden-and-build theory of positive emotions. *Philosophical Transactions of the Royal Society, 359,* 1367–1377. Wadlinger, H., & Isaacowitz, D. (2006). Positive mood broadens visual attention to positive stimuli. *Motivation and Emotion, 30*(1), 87–99.

"The one you feed": This parable has over 200 online entries and it's origin is unclear. Retrieved September 25, 2008, from *blog.beliefnet.com/jwalking/2007/03/ cherokee-wisdom.html.*

Research shows that expressing anger: Bushman, B. (2002). Does venting anger feed or extinguish the flame?: Catharsis, rumination, distraction, anger and aggressive responding. *Personality and Social Psychology Bulletin, 28*(6), 724–731. Lewis, W., & Bucher, A. (1992). Anger, catharsis, the reformulated frustration–aggression hypothesis, and health consequences. *Psychotherapy: Theory, Research, Practice, Training, 29*(3), 385–392.

Between these two my life flows: Nisargadatta Maharaj, Dikshit, S., & Frydman, M. (2000). *I am that: Talks with Sri Nisargadatta* (p. 269). Durham, NC: Acorn Press.

Selfing and the Brain: Farb, N., Segal, Z., Mayberg, H., Beau, J., McKeon, D., Fatima, Z., & Anderson, A. (2007). Attending to the present: Mindfulness meditation reveals distinct neural modes of self-reference. *Social Cognitive and Affective Neuroscience, 2*(4), 313–322.

overall happiness level: Lyubomirsky, S., Sheldon, K., & Schkade, D. (2005). Pursuing happiness: The architecture of sustainable change. *Review of General Psychology, 9*(2), 111–131.

"attachment theory": Wallin, D. (2007). *Attachment in psychotherapy.* New York: Guilford Press.

We also *internalize* images of caregivers: Summers, F. (1994). *Object relations theories and psychopathology: A comprehensive text.* New York: Analytic Press/Taylor & Francis Group.

CHAPTER 6. CARING FOR OURSELVES

I have great faith in a seed: Thoreau, H. (1993). *Faith in a seed* (quote in front matter). Washington, DC: Island Press.

translation of the Pali word *metta*: Buddharakkhita, A. (1989/1995). Metta: The philosophy and practice of universal love. *Buddhist Publication Society/Access to Insight edition.* Accessed September 27, 2008, from *www.accesstoinsight.org/lib/authors/buddharakkhita/wheel365.html.* Rhys Davids, T., & Stede, W. (1921/2001). *Pali-English Dictionary* (p. 540). New Delhi: Munishiram Manoharlal.

instructions for cultivating loving-kindness: Buddhaghosa, B., & Nanamoli, B. (1975). The divine abidings. In *The path of purification: Visuddhimagga* (pp. 321–353). Kandy, Sri Lanka: Buddhist Publication Society.

May all beings be happy and secure: From the *Metta Sutta, Sutta Nipata* 145–151, translated October 2, 2008, by Andrew Olendzki, Executive Director of the Barre Center for Buddhist Studies, Barre, MA.

the first person to introduce metta meditation: Salzberg, S. (1995). *Lovingkindness: The revolutionary art of happiness.* Boston: Shambhala.

against the repressive government of Myanmar: Senauke, H. (2008, Summer). Grace under pressure. *Buddhadharma: The Practitioner's Quarterly,* pp. 56–63.

Compassion Meditation and the Brain: Lutz, A., Greischar, L., Rawlings, N., Richard, M., & Davidson, R. (2004). Long-term meditators self-induce high-amplitude gamma synchrony during mental practice. *Proceedings of the National Academy of Science, 101*(46), 16369–16373. Lutz, A., Brefczynski-Lewis, J., Johnstone, T., & Davidson, R. (2008). Regulation of the neural circuitry of emotion by compassion meditation: Effects of meditative expertise. *PLoS ONE, 3*(3): e1897. Accessed December 18, 2008, from *www.plosone.org/article/info:doi/10.1371/journal.pone.0001897.*

lack of self-compassion is not a unique quality of Western life: Neff, K., Pisitsungkagarn, K., & Hseih, Y. (2008). Self-compassion and self-construal in the United States, Thailand, and Taiwan. *Journal of Cross-Cultural Psychology, 39,* 267–285.

disciple asks the rebbe: Moyers, W., & Ketcham, K. (2006). In *Broken: My story of addiction and redemption* (front matter, from *The politics of the brokenhearted* by Parker J. Palmer). New York: Viking Press.

Loving-Kindness Builds Positive Resources: Fredrickson, B., Cohn, M., Coffey, K., Pek, J., & Finkel, S. (2008). Open hearts build lives: Positive emotions, induced through loving-kindness meditation, build consequential personal resources. *Journal of Personality and Social Psychology, 95*(5), 1045–1062. McCorkle, B. (2008, August). *The relationship between compassion and wisdom: Experimental observations and reflections.* Paper presented at the annual convention of the American Psychological Association, Boston, MA. A pilot study of loving-kindness meditation (15 min. 4×/week for 5 weeks) shifted views of oneself and "difficult persons" from fault-finding to broader understanding of the complexities of behavior.

stay close to the *wishing* side: Retrieved December 17, 2007, from *groups.yahoo. com/group/giftoflovingkindness.*

Attend to your sensitivity: Mead, D. (2008). If you would grow to your best self. Poem retrieved September 20, 2008, from *www.balancedweightmanagement.com/IfYou-WouldGrow.htm.*

When Prayer Is Avoidance: Zettle, R., Hocker, T., Mick, K., Scofield, B., Petersen, C., Song, H., et al. (2005). Differential strategies in coping with pain as a function of the level of experiential avoidance. *Psychological Record, 55*(4), 511–524.

The bud stands for all things: Kinnell, G. (1980). Saint Francis and the sow. In W. H. Roetzheim (Ed.). (2006). *The giant book of poetry* (p. 484). Jamul, CA: Level4-Press.

Before you know kindness as the deepest thing inside: Nye, N. (1995). Kindness. In *Words under the words* (pp. 42–43). Portland, OR: Eighth Mountain Press.

Loving-Kindness Meditation Reduces Back Pain: Carson, J., Keefe, F., Lynch, T., Carson, K., Goli, V., Fras, A., & Thorp, S. (2005). Loving-kindness meditation for chronic low back pain. *Journal of Holistic Nursing, 23*(3), 287–304.

So, when the shoe fits: Merton, T. (1965). *The way of Chuang Tzu* (p. 112). New York: New Directions.

CHAPTER 7. CARING FOR OTHERS

High levels of compassion: Davidson, R., & Harrington, A. (2002). *Visions of compassion: Western scientists and Tibetan Buddhists examine human nature.* Oxford, UK: Oxford University Press, p. 98.

"People are a problem": Adams, D. (2002). In *The ultimate hitchhiker's guide to the galaxy* (p. 278). New York: Del Rey.

"Hatred corrodes the vessel in which it's stored": Chinese proverb. Retrieved October 1, 2008, from *www.worldofquotes.com/author/Proverb/94/index.html.*

Looking after oneself, one looks after others: Olendzki, A. (2005). Sedaka sutta: The bamboo acrobat. Translated from the Pali by A. Olendzki, *Access to Insight.* Retrieved December 14, 2008, from *www.accesstoinsight.org/tipitaka/sn/sn47/sn47.019. olen.html.*

connection has an ebb and a flow: Surrey, J. (2005). Relational psychotherapy, relational mindfulness. In C. Germer, R. Siegel, & P. Fulton (Eds.), *Mindfulness and psychotherapy* (pp. 91–112). New York: Guilford Press.

"the things you cannot see": Carter, J. (1998). *The things you cannot see.* Commencement address at the University of Pennsylvania. Retrieved October 1, 2008, from *www.upenn.edu/almanac/v44/n34/98gradspeeches.html.* The entire quote is: "Two thousand years ago, the people of Corinth asked St. Paul this question: 'What is the most important thing of all?' The way they expressed it was, 'What are the things in human life that never change?' And Paul gave a strange answer. He said, 'They're the things you cannot see.' You can see money, you can see a house, you can see your name in the paper. What are the things you cannot see that should be paramount in our lives? You can't see justice, peace, service, humility. You can't see forgiveness, compassion and, if you will excuse the expression, love."

there is a cloud floating in this sheet of paper: Nhat Hanh, T. (1991). In *Peace is every step* (p. 95). New York: Bantam Books.

60 million Americans suffer from loneliness: Cacioppo, J., & Patrick, W. (2008). *Loneliness: Human nature and the need for social connection.* New York: Norton.

lonelier than their counterparts in Spain: Rokach, A., Moya, M., Orzeck, T., & Exposito, F. (2001). Loneliness in North America and Spain. *Social Behavior and Personality, 29*(5), 477–489.

the trustworthiness of others: Rahm, W., & Transue, J. (1998). Social trust and value change: The decline of social capital in American youth, 1976–1995. *Political Psychology, 19*(3), 545–565.

"nomadic society on this treadmill": DeAngelis, T. (2007, April). America: Toxic lifestyle? *Monitor on Psychology,* pp. 50–52.

If you wish to make an apple pie from scratch: Sagan, C. (2002). In *New ideas about new ideas: Insights on creativity from the world's leading innovators* (p. 268), by S. White & G. Wright. Cambridge, MA: DaCapo Press.

The building blocks for empathizing with other people: Rizzolatti, G., Sinigaglia, C., & Anderson, F. (2008). *Mirrors in the brain: How our minds share actions, emotions, and experience.* London: Oxford University Press. Goleman, D. (2006). *Social intelligence: The new science of human relationships.* New York: Bantam Books. Siegel, D. (2007). *The mindful brain: Reflections and attunement in the cultivation of well-being.* New York: Norton. Dobbs, D. (2006, April–May). A revealing connection. *Scientific American Mind,* pp. 22–27.

A human being is part of the whole called by us "universe": Einstein, A. (1972, March 29). *New York Times.* In J. Austin (1999), *Zen and the brain* (p. 652). Cambridge, MA: MIT Press.

"He's just not that into you!": Behrendt, G., Tuccillo, L., & Monchik, L. (2006). *He's just not that into you: The no-excuses truth to understanding guys.* New York: Simon Spotlight Entertainment.

Metta Changes the Brain, Making Us More Compassionate: Davidson, R. (2007, October 20). *Changing the brain by transforming the mind: The impact of compassion* *training on the neural systems of emotion.* Paper presented at the Mind and Life Institute Conference, Investigating the Mind: Mindfulness, Compassion, and the Treatment of Depression, with His Holiness the Dalai Lama, Emory University, Atlanta, GA.

Loving-Kindness toward Strangers: Hutcherson, C., Seppala, E., & Gross, J. (2008). Loving-kindness meditation increases social connectedness. *Emotion, 8*(5), 720–724.

Compassion Fatigue: Rothschild, B., & Rand, M. (2006). *Help for the helper: The psychophysiology of compassion fatigue and vicarious trauma.* New York: Norton.

People seek happiness in three different ways: Seligman, M. (2002). *Authentic happiness: Using the new positive psychology to realize your potential for lasting fulfillment.* New York: Free Press. Sirgy, M., & Wu, J. (2007, September). The pleasant life, the engaged life, and the meaningful life: What about the balanced life? *Journal of Happiness Studies,* DOI 10.1007/s10902-9074-1. Retrieved October 1, 2008, from *www. springerlink.com/content/j0572642qk126014/*.

acute lymphoblastic leukemia: Henderson, J. (2008, March/April). Blindsided. *Psychotherapy Networker, 32*(2), 50–56.

CHAPTER 8. FINDING YOUR BALANCE

Man always travels along precipices: Gonzales, P. (2007). In *Ortega's "The revolt of the masses" and the triumph of the new man* (p. 67). New York: Algora. From Ortega, J. (1956). In *The dehumanization of art and other writings on art and culture* (p. 189). New York: Doubleday.

a method of overcoming suffering: Ribush, N. (Ed.). (2005). In *Teachings from Tibet: Guidance from great lamas* (pp. 173–174). Weston, MA: Lama Yeshe Wisdom Archive. This quote is the Dalai Lama's paraphrase of a verse of the 8th-century sage, Shantideva:

> If something can be remedied
> Why be unhappy about it?
> And if there is not remedy for it,
> There is still no point in being unhappy.

Kelsang Gyatso, G., & Elliott, N. (2002). In *Guide to the bodhisattva's way of life: A Buddhist poem for today* (p. 70, chapter 6, verse 10). Glen Spey, NY: Tharpa.

"The intellect is a good servant but a poor master": Surya Das, L. (2008). In *Words of wisdom* (p. 133). Kihei, HI: Koa Books.

Perfectionism begins in childhood: Flett, G., & Hewett, P. (2002). *Perfectionism: Theory, research, and treatment.* Washington, DC: American Psychological Association. Blatt, S. (1995). The destructiveness of perfectionism: Implications for the treatment of depression. *American Psychologist, 50*(12), 1003–1020. Pacht, A. (1984). Reflections on perfection. *American Psychologist, 39*(4), 386–390.

"trance of unworthiness": Brach, T. (2003). *Radical acceptance: Embracing your life with the heart of a Buddha.* New York: Bantam Dell.

work more than 50 hours a week: International Labor Organization statistics, reported by Alan Hedge, professor of design and environmental analysis at Cornell University, in DeAngelis, T. (2007, April). America: Toxic lifestyle? In *Monitor on Psychology.* Washington, DC: American Psychological Association.

the self-improvement industry is worth over $9.6 billion annually: Market-data Enterprises, Inc. (2006, September 1). The US market for self-improvement products and services. Retrieved September 20, 2008, from *www.marketresearch.com/product/display.asp?productid=1338280&g=1.*

cost to their health and relationships: Banks, J., Marmot, M., Oldfield, Z., & Smith, J. (2006). Disease and disadvantage in the United States and in England. *Journal of the American Medical Association, 295*(17), 2037–2045.

the creative dedicated minority has made the world better: King, M. (1981). In *Strength to love* (p. 61). Minneapolis, MN: Fortress Press.

nothing harder than the softness of indifference: Robertson, C. (Ed.). (1998). In *Dictionary of quotations* (p. 293). Hertfordshire, UK: Wordsworth Editions.

"Half the world knows not how the other half lives": Smith, W., & Heseltine, J. (Eds.). (1936). In *The Oxford dictionary of English proverbs* (p. 128). Oxford, UK: Clarendon Press.

"Extraverts" are gregarious, generally happy people/"introverts" enjoy the inner life: Laney, M. (2002). *The introvert advantage: How to thrive in an extrovert world.* New York: Workman. Wikipedia, the free encyclopedia. (2008, September 22). *Extraversion and introversion.* Retrieved September 22, 2008, from *en.wikipedia. org/wiki/Extroversion.*

genetic and brain differences may partially account for the differences: Tellegen, A., Lykken, D., Bouchard, T., Wilcox, K., Segal, N., & Rich, S. (1988). Personality similarity in twins reared apart and together. *Journal of Personality and Social Psychology, 54*(6), 1031–1039. Depue, R., & Collins, P. (1999). Neurobiology of the structure of personality: Dopamine, facilitation of incentive motivation, and extraversion. *Behavioral and Brain Sciences, 22,* 491–517. Johnson, D., Wiebe, J., Gold, S., & Andreasen, N. (1999). Cerebral blood flow and personality: A positron emission tomography study. *American Journal of Psychiatry, 156,* 252–257.

the five mental "hindrances": Brahmavamso, A. (1999, April). The five hindrances (*Nivarana*). *Buddhist Society of Western Australia Newsletter.* Retrieved October 1, 2008, from *mail.saigon.com/~anson/ebud/ebmed051.htm.*

The fastest progress ... is achieved by those who are content: Brahmavamso, A. (1999, April). The five hindrances (*Nivarana*)/Restlessness. *Buddhist Society of Western Australia Newsletter.* Retrieved October 1, 2008, from *mail.saigon.com/~anson/ebud/ebmed051.htm.*

mindfulness-based relapse prevention: Witkiewitz, K., Marlatt, G., & Walker, D. (2005). Mindfulness-based relapse prevention for alcohol and substance use disorders. *Journal of Cognitive Psychotherapy: An International Quarterly, 19*(3), 211–228.

spiritual self-schema therapy: Margolin, A., Schuman-Olivier, Z., Beitel, M., Arnold, R., Fulwiler, C., & Avants, S. (2007). A preliminary study of spiritual self-schema (3-S⁺) therapy for reducing impulsivity in HIV-positive drug users. *Journal of Clinical Psychology, 63*(10), 979–989. Beitel, M., Genove, M., Schuman-Olivier, Z., Arnold, R., Avants, S., & Margolin, A. (2007). Reflections by inner-city drug users on a Buddhist-based spirituality-focused therapy: A qualitative study. *American Journal of Orthopsychiatry, 77*(1), 1–9. Avants, S., & Margolin, A. (2004). Development of spiritual self-schema (3-S) therapy for the treatment of addictive and HIV risk behavior: A convergence of cognitive and Buddhist psychology. *Journal of Psychotherapy Integration, 14*(3), 253–289. Margolin, A., Beitel, M., Schuman-Olivier, Z., & Avants, S. (2006). A controlled study of a spiritually-focused intervention for increasing motivation for HIV prevention among drug users. *AIDS Education and Prevention, 18*(4), 311–322.

CHAPTER 9. MAKING PROGRESS

Suffering doesn't disappear from our life: Magid, B. (2008). In *Ending the pursuit of happiness: A Zen guide* (p. 70). Somerville, MA: Wisdom Publications.

leave the doctors and nurses to talk to the sickness: Brahm, A. (2005). In J. Bartok (Ed.), *More daily wisdom* (p. 139). Somerville, MA: Wisdom. Originally in Brahm, A. (2003). *Who ordered this truckload of dung?: Inspiring stories for welcoming life's difficulties.* Somerville, MA: Wisdom.

Stages of Self-Compassion: Morgan, W. (1991). Change in meditation: A phenomenological study of Vipassana meditator's views of progress. *Dissertation Abstracts International, 51*(7-B), 3575–3576. This doctoral thesis identified four stages of meditation practice: striving, disappointment, reevaluation, and acceptance. For similar stages, see pp. 11–14 in Magid, B. (2008). *Ending the pursuit of happiness: A Zen guide.* Somerville, MA: Wisdom.

"All techniques are destined to fail!": Smith, R. (2006, January 12). From a talk at the Mind and Life Institute Scientist's Retreat at the Insight Meditation Society, Barre, MA.

a model of psychotherapy based on core values and commitments: Hayes, S., & Smith, S. (2005). *Get out of your mind and into your life: The new acceptance and commitment therapy.* Oakland, CA: New Harbinger. Hayes, S., Strosahl, K., & Wilson, K. (1999). *Acceptance and commitment therapy: An experimental approach to behavior change.* New York: Guilford Press.

"Neurons that fire together, wire together": Hebb, D. (1949). *The organization of behavior: A neuropsychological theory.* New York: Bantam Books.

"What would your best friend say to you right now?": Roth, B. (2008). Family dharma: Befriending yourself. *Tricycle: The Buddhist Review.* Retrieved October 1, 2008, from *www.tricycle.com/web_exclusive/3698-1.html.*

engage your children: Goodman, T., & Greenland, S. (2008). Mindfulness with children: Working with difficult emotions (pp. 415–429). In F. Didonna (Ed.), *Clinical handbook of mindfulness.* New York: Springer. The authors suggest an acronym for children, S-C-R-A-M, as an antidote to running away from difficult emotions: Stop or slow down, Calm your body, Remember to look at what's happening, take Action with Metta (act with kindness).

"gleam of the particulars": Nye, N. (1995). *Words under the words: Selected poems* (back cover). Portland, OR: Eighth Mountain Press.

tough attitude toward our emotions: A study of experienced paramedics in Austria found that well-being was correlated with having "contempt" and "tough control" over one's feelings ("ignoring one's own emotions to serve others … as long as helping doesn't overly tax the helper"). Future research will probably explore the conditions (social norms, survival, need for control) and long-term outcomes of "successful nonacceptance" of emotion. Mitmansgruber, H., Beck, T., & Schussler, G. (2008). "Mindful helpers": Experiential avoidance, meta-emotions, and emotion regulation in paramedics. *Journal of Research in Personality, 42,* 1358–1363.

"We can still be crazy after all these years": Chödrön, P. (1991/2001): *The wisdom of no escape and the path of loving-kindness* (p. 4). Boston: Shambhala.

APPENDIX A. EMOTION WORDS

Emotion Words: DeRose, S. (2005, July 6). *The compass DeRose guide to emotion words.* Retrieved October 6, 2008, from *www.derose.net/steve/resources/emotionwords/ewords.html.* Reprinted by permission of Steven J. DeRose.

APPENDIX B. ADDITIONAL SELF-COMPASSION EXERCISES

Giving and taking meditation is attributed to: Tharchin, S. (1999). *Achieving bodhichitta: Instructions of two great lineages combined into a unique system of eleven categories* (pp. 63–98). Howell, NJ: Mahayana Sutra and Tantra Press.

When the Dalai Lama was asked how he meditates: Dalai Lama & Chan, V. (2004). *The wisdom of forgiveness: Intimate conversations and journeys* (pp. 73–74). New York: Riverhead Books.

Centering became popular: Pennington, B. (1982). *Centering Prayer: Renewing an ancient Christian prayer form.* Garden City, NY: Image Books.

Light a candle and place it before you: This meditation is adapted from the light (*jyoti*) meditation taught by Satya Sai Baba of Puttaparthi, India. Retrieved September 15, 2008, from *www.saibaba.ws/teachings/jyotimeditation.htm.*

"A flower touches everyone's heart": Drohojowska-Philp, H. (2004). In *Full bloom: The art and life of Georgia O'Keefe* (p. 380). New York: Norton.

"my senses put in tune once more": In R. Finch & J. Elder (Eds.). (1990). *The Norton book of nature writing* (p. 274). New York: Norton. The entire quote is: "When I go to town, my ear suffers as well as my nose: the impact of the city upon my senses is hard and dissonant; the ear is stunned, the nose is outraged, and the eye is confused. When I come back, I go to Nature to be soothed and healed, and to have my senses put in tune once more."

compassionate guide to nature meditation: Coleman, M. (2006). *Awake in the wild: Mindfulness in nature as a path of self-discovery.* Novato, CA: New World Library.

one of the Dalai Lama's favorite vows: Dalai Lama, with Piburn, S. (Ed.). (1990). The Nobel Peace Prize Lecture. In *The Dalai Lama: A Policy of Kindness* (p. 27). Ithaca, NY: Snow Lion.

index

about the author

Christopher K. Germer, PhD, is a clinical psychologist in private practice, specializing in mindfulness- and acceptance-based treatment. He has been integrating the principles and practices of meditation into psychotherapy since 1978 and has taken numerous journeys to India to explore the varieties of meditation. Dr. Germer is a Clinical Instructor in Psychology at Harvard Medical School and a founding member of the Institute for Meditation and Psychotherapy, an organization dedicated to teaching mental health professionals how to integrate ancient Buddhist psychology into effective modern psychotherapy. He lectures internationally on mindfulness and self-compassion. Dr. Germer is a codeveloper with Kristin Neff of the 8-week Mindful Self-Compassion training, and coeditor of the professionally acclaimed books *Mindfulness and Psychotherapy* and *Wisdom and Compassion in Psychotherapy*.